Diabetes

RECIPES

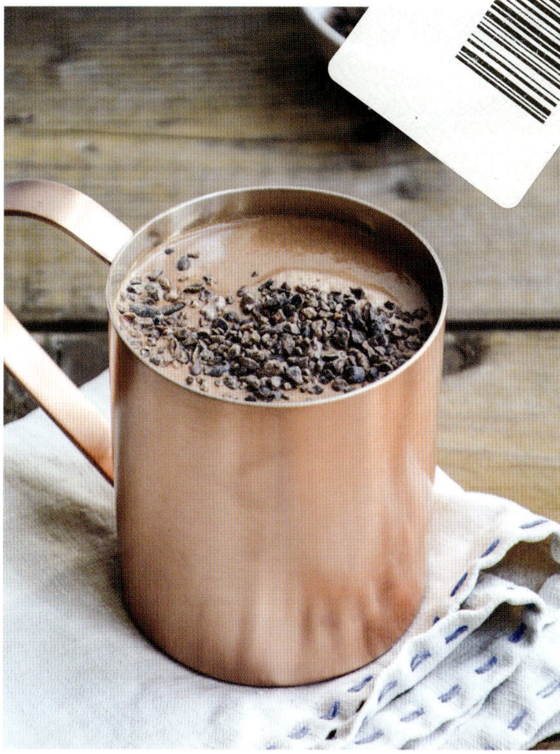

JESS LOMAS

WP

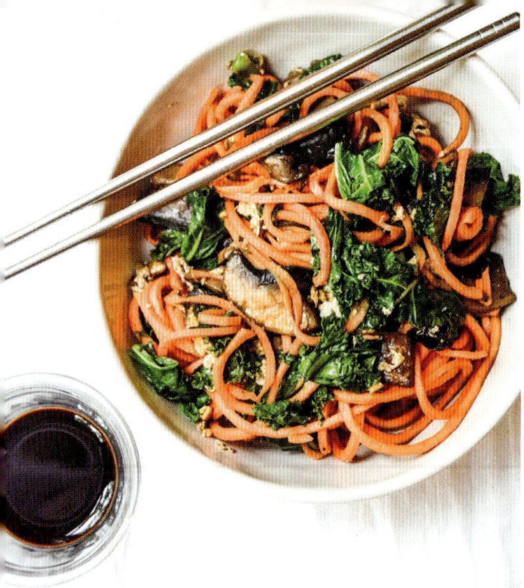

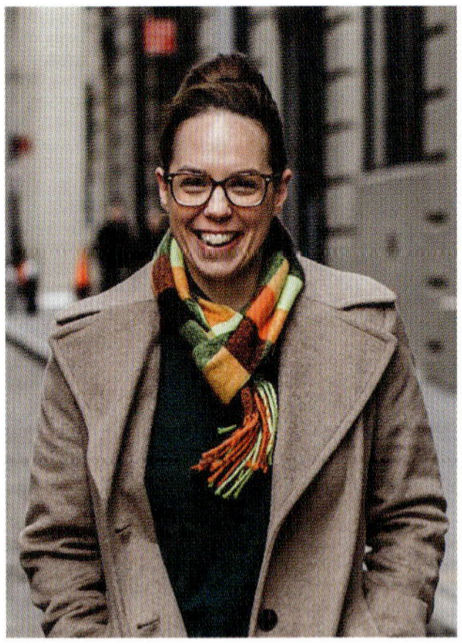

JESS LOMAS is an author and editor from Melbourne, Australia. Her previous titles include *Real Food Treats, Real Food Kids, Low Sugar – Collected Edition, Sugar Detox* and *Diabetes – Collected Edition*. Follow her on Instagram or Twitter @jesslomas.

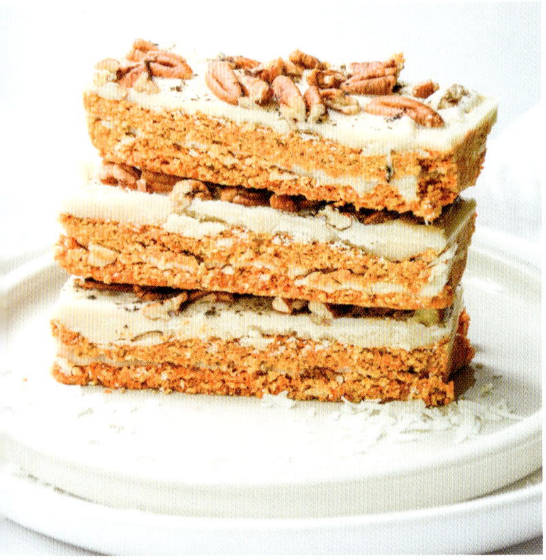

Published by:
Wilkinson Publishing Pty Ltd
ACN 006 042 173
Level 4, 2 Collins St Melbourne, Victoria, Australia 3000
Ph: +61 3 9654 5446
www.wilkinsonpublishing.com.au

Creator: Lomas, Jess, author.

Title: Diabetes recipes : healthy ideas for balancing blood sugar /Jess Lomas.

ISBN: 9781925642209 (paperback)

Subjects: Diabetes--Diet therapy--Recipes.
Cooking.
Sugar--Health aspects.
Food--Sugar content.
Sugar-free diet--Recipes.

Photos and illustrations by agreement with photo agencies including Getty.
Recipe photography by agreement with Jess Lomas.

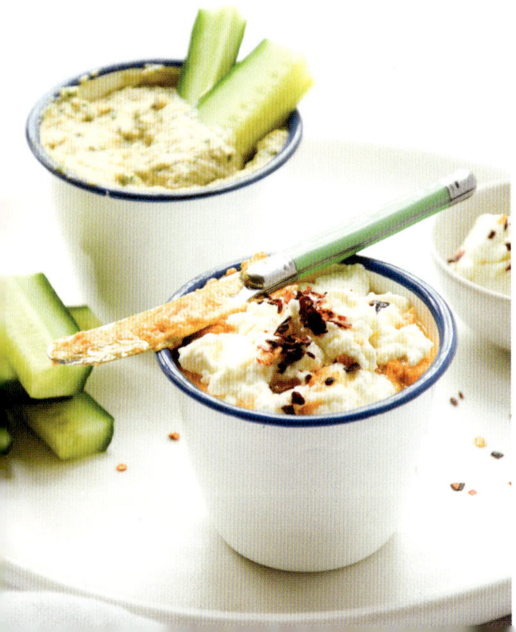

contents

Introduction 4
What is diabetes? 6
Saturated fat: friend or foe? 9
The Low-carb question 12
Diabetes, heart disease & omega 3s 15
Low Sugar Living 17
Ditch the drinks 22
Does size matter? 24
Top foods to stabilise blood sugar 28
Stress & Diabetes: A match made in heaven 30
Breakfasts 34
Salads & sides 52
Mains 86
Drinks 121
Treats 142
Recipe index 160

Introduction

IT'S BEEN THREE YEARS since the first edition of *Diabetes Recipes* was released and unfortunately the diabetes epidemic has only continued to grow. Now more than ever it's important to spread the message of this book and share the recipes for healthy living. Whether you have been diagnosed with diabetes yourself or know someone who has, it's not too late to take control of your health and wellbeing. With tips on stress relief, portion control and top foods to stabilise blood sugar levels, this guide also has healthy, delicious recipes for you to dip into daily for inspiration and encouragement. The diagnosis of diabetes can be a scary and confusing time, not just for the diagnosed individual but also for their family. Suddenly food is not just for fuel or pleasure but something that can put your very life in danger as you learn how to navigate the blood sugar maze.

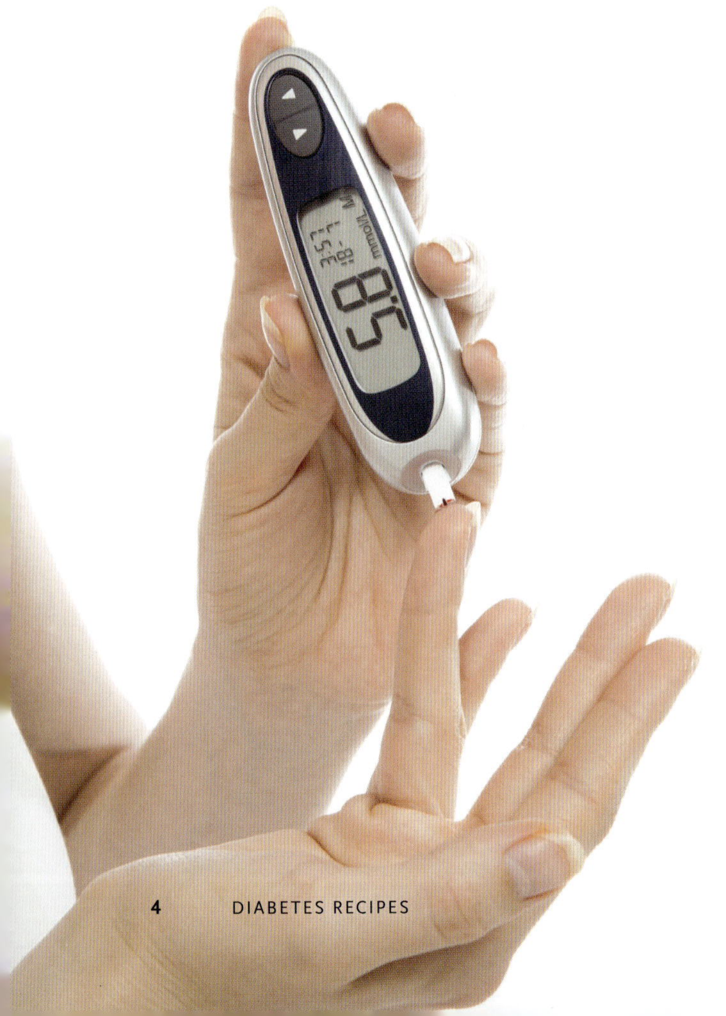

This new edition of *Diabetes Recipes* combines some **much-loved recipes** from previous editions with new and exciting ideas to revitalise your menu plan and help balance your blood sugar. It was several years ago now that a member of my own family came face to face with a diabetes diagnosis.

My understanding of diabetes comes from loving a person who has type 2, and not from experiencing it myself. I do not know what it feels like to have to check my blood glucose multiple times a day, nor the feeling of having to use medication such as insulin. I also don't know what it feels like to have numbness in my feet or a blood sugar spike after eating something I thought would be okay. Despite this, I do know what it feels like to walk into a supermarket and stare at the abundance on offer and think: what should I be feeding my body? And I understand the thinking behind, and stress that can sometimes arise, from cooking a meal for a friend or loved one with diabetes, not wanting them to miss out but also wanting to do the best for them and their body.

After the diagnosis in my family, I stopped and took stock of my own diet and lifestyle. **Type 2 diabetes does not come about overnight;** it is a result of, sometimes, a lifetime of bad habit building blocks crashing down. Other times, as we are seeing more frequently today, it is occurring in younger people as a result of ambushing developing bodies with incorrect sustenance. Of course we must be aware of the genetic elements that come into play, but we cannot solely blame genetics when we are also leading stressful and more sedentary lives while consuming increased amounts of highly processed foods that put our bodies under strain.

As a result of taking the time to look to the future, I decided to try and **reduce my chances** of developing type 2 diabetes later in life by changing my lifestyle now. I heavily reduced the amount of sugar in my diet, in turn reducing the overall amount of processed food I was consuming. **Removing excess sugar** in your diet forces you to get back in the kitchen and create amazing, healthy meals from scratch.

People with diabetes should not feel that they cannot enjoy food the way they used to or that they cannot indulge from time to time like a person without diabetes might; but they do have an inescapable reason to educate themselves about their own health and what they can do to get the most out of their body and their life.

As with any health topic there is an abundance of **contradictory information** available about causes, triggers, treatments and cures. Type 2 diabetes is no different, and while the following is in no way medical advice to replace that of your regular physician, it is an alternative view to the mainstream thinking. It is important to note that no one diet or lifestyle suits

> People with diabetes should not feel that they cannot enjoy food the way they used to

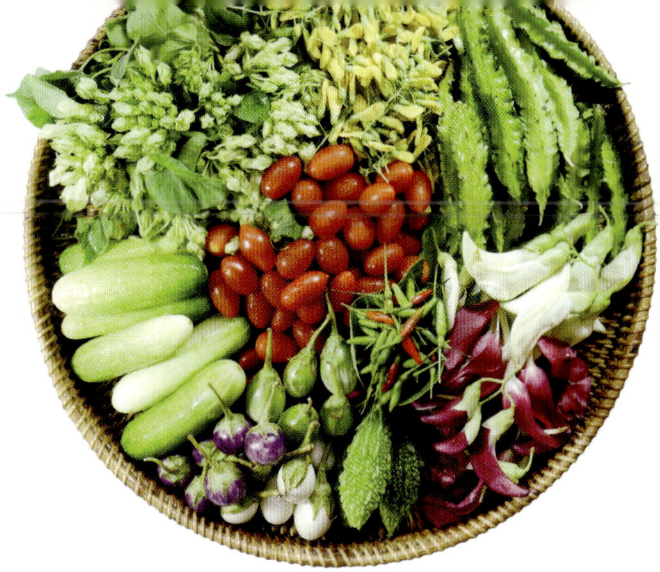

everyone equally. What works for you might not work for the next person, and so **personal responsibility** becomes important when knowing what foods trigger blood glucose spikes and what foods are "safe" specifically for you.

It is worth your time to **research your condition** further beyond what your doctor may tell you while prescribing you medication. Medication is indispensable in treating diabetes, especially during the early stages of diagnosis. However, as with any illness or disease there is room to incorporate alternative or natural treatments alongside your medication to treat your body as a whole and not just the symptoms of the disease. Nourishing your entire body by feeding it whole foods, managing stress and leading an active lifestyle has proven to be beneficial for so many in their diabetes management.

Diabetes Recipes is primarily concerned with type 2 diabetes, as this is **influenced more by lifestyle** and is the epidemic sweeping the world, sustained by concerning figures of overweight and obesity. Somewhere along the way we've become lost, trusting our health to corporations and the packaged foods they provide for us or the medication their profits depend on. It's time to take our health and happiness back into our own hands, roll up our sleeves and get back into the kitchen to prepare wholesome meals that can fuel our bodies and keep the symptoms of diabetes under control.

What is diabetes?

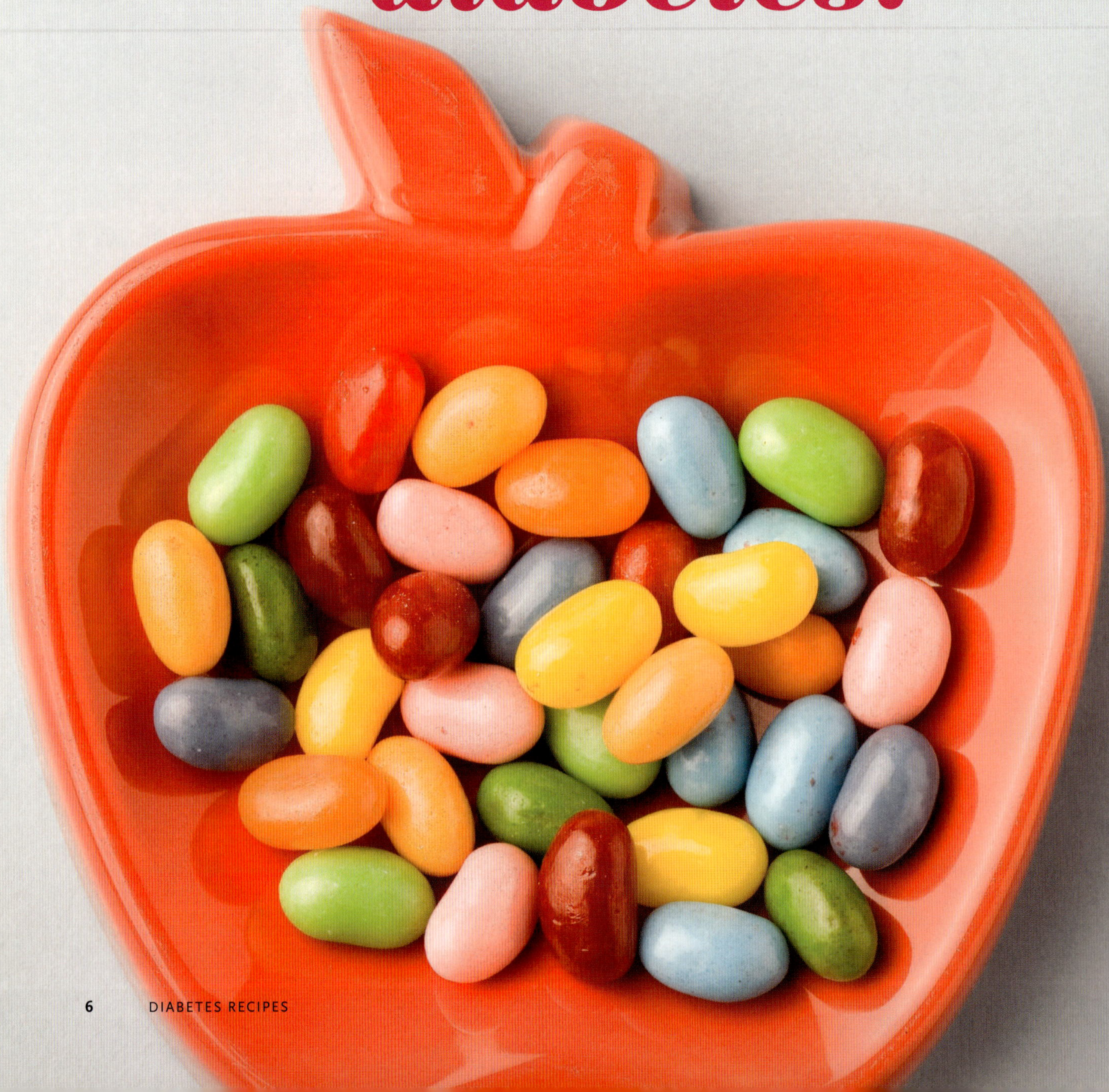

TYPE 2 DIABETES was once referred to as adult-onset diabetes or non-insulin dependent diabetes. It can no longer be called adult-onset diabetes as it is non-discriminatory against age, affecting children and teenagers as well as adults.

Type 2 diabetes occurs when your **body is unable to produce insulin sufficiently** and is unable to regulate the amount of glucose in the blood. As with many diseases, the body's ability to cope with the symptoms of diabetes decreases with age and the length of diagnosis if the individual doesn't manage their condition appropriately.

Glucose is our body's primary source of fuel. When we eat food, the pancreas releases insulin to help the body absorb glucose from the blood into our muscle tissues for fuel and cellular respiration, while the liver, which stores glucose, releases more. **Insulin** is vital to the body, ensuring there isn't an excess build up of glucose in the blood, which can lead to insulin resistance, a predecessor to type 2 diabetes. Insulin resistance forces your pancreas to produce more and more insulin to try and regulate your blood glucose levels. As any machine working on overdrive eventually does, your pancreas soon can't keep up with the demands and blood glucose levels rise, resulting in **type 2 diabetes**. As a result of this process your pancreas can no longer produce the **correct amount** of insulin and your body reacts differently to the consumption of food, especially **high carbohydrate foods** or foods **high in sugar**. It can also mean your body is less stable than a non-diabetic's during periods of fasting, such as between meals, when your blood glucose levels can drop suddenly.

The body's ability to cope with the symptoms of diabetes decreases with age and length of diagnosis

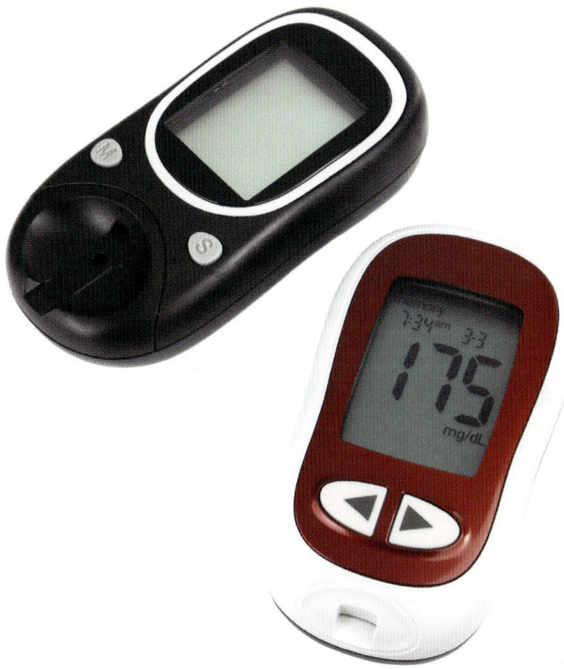

Diabetes Australia suggests that up to **60% of diabetes cases** could have been delayed or prevented through a combination of physical activity, maintaining a healthy weight, not smoking and managing blood pressure and cholesterol. Once you have been given the diabetes diagnosis, your **risk increases for complications** including stroke, heart attack or heart disease, kidney damage, gangrene and amputation of the feet, and even blindness. This makes management of your condition a high priority for quality of life.

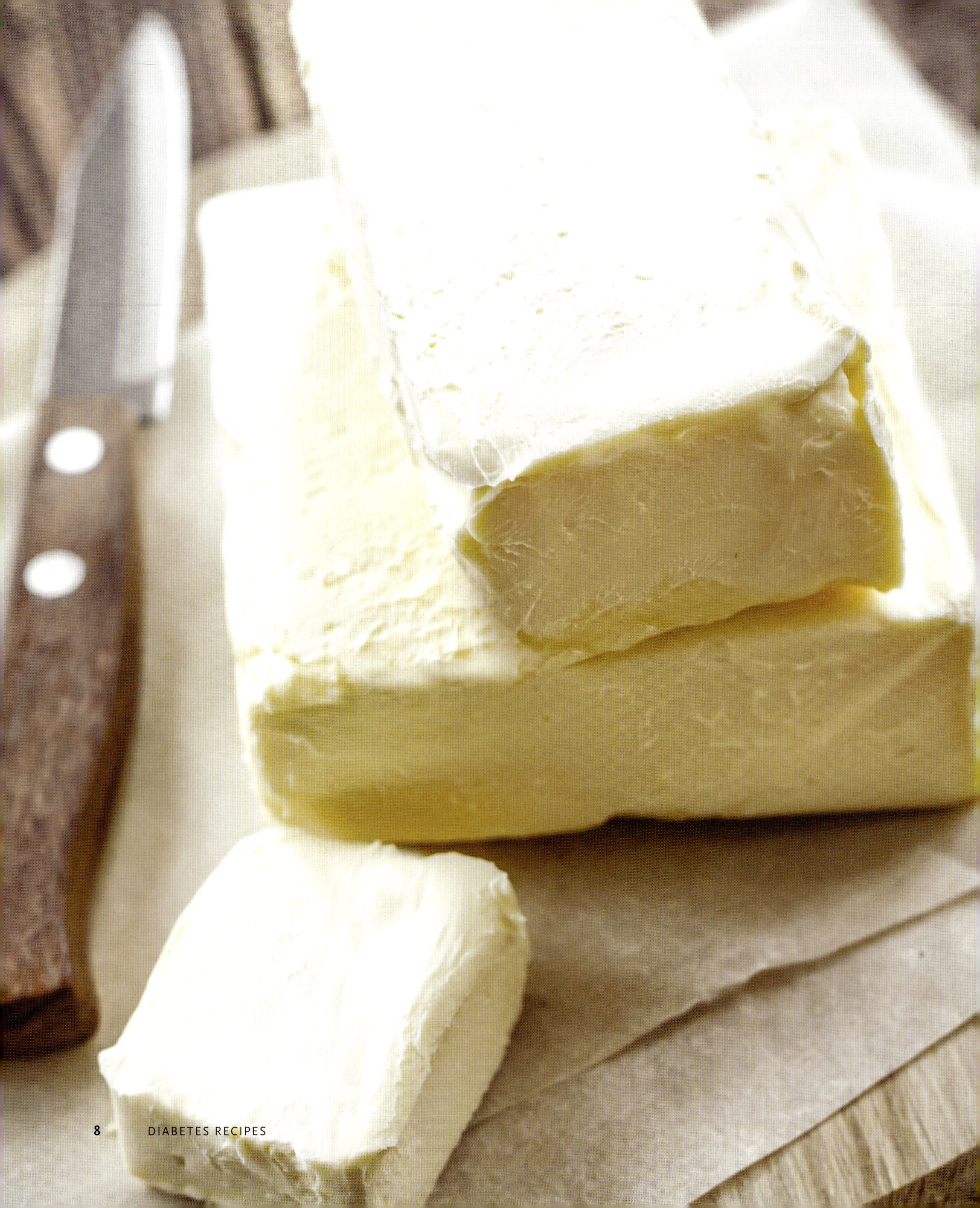

Saturated fat:

friend or foe?

HERE'S WHERE READERS may become divided. The traditional way of thinking, at least since the 1970s, is that saturated fat should be minimised in the diet or better yet, avoided entirely. This is the mantra you'll hear from various diabetes and heart associations around the world: saturated fat, found in animal products such as meat and full fat milk and cheese, will raise your LDL "bad" cholesterol and accelerate weight gain. Their thinking is that fat makes you fat, and excess weight and elevated cholesterol levels make excess glucose in the blood harder to manage, leading to insulin resistance, diabetes and diabetes complications.

In the article *Saturated fat is not the major issue* from the *British Medical Journal* dated October 22, 2013, interventional cardiology specialist registrar Aseem Malhotra wrote that, "the mantra that saturated fat **must be removed** to reduce the risk of cardiovascular disease has dominated dietary advice and guidelines for almost four decades.

"Yet scientific evidence shows that this advice has, paradoxically, increased our cardiovascular risks ... Saturated fat has been demonised ever since Ansel Keys's landmark "seven countries" study in 1970. This concluded that a correlation existed between the incidence of coronary heart disease and total cholesterol concentrations, which then correlated with the proportion of energy provided by saturated fat. But correlation is not causation."

At the time there were two schools of thought competing for mainstream recognition: Ansel Keys, who believed that **saturated fat** was our **biggest enemy**, and John Yudkin, who believed **refined sugar** was more responsible for many illnesses, including heart disease. In the decades that have passed since Keys released his findings, incidence of heart disease and obesity have not reduced in line with the dietary changes. Over the years, as we've removed saturated fat we've also increased our sugar consumption as we pump more of it into products that don't need it. In turn, **diabetes has become an epidemic**, heart disease is still one of the largest killers, and chronic disease is affecting more and more people. What this could lead you to question is the bigger picture, rather than isolating saturated fat as the sole enemy.

Over the years, as we've removed saturated fat we've also increased our sugar consumption

Our brains need **good quality fats** to function optimally, but along the line we have become confused by what constitutes a *good* fat and what is a *bad* fat. Over the years saturated fat and trans fat have been lumped together as the fats to avoid, while monounsaturated fats and polyunsaturated fats have been given the green tick. It's quite confusing when attempting to decide what's good to eat and what to avoid.

When deciding to remove or reduce saturated fat from the diet, alternative foods have been produced to feed those looking for a **"healthier"** alternative. Margarine has replaced butter; full fat milk and cheese have been ditched for low-fat options (where the fat is taken out and replaced with various ingredients including sugar, so the product still tastes good), and in place of coconut oil we have been told to use vegetable and seed oils such as canola. The bottom line is: we have been replacing *real* food with **manmade, manufactured products** that are created in a lab or a factory rather than grown or reared on the land.

In his book, *Toxic Oil*, author David Gillespie says, "There is no evidence that saturated fats cause **heart disease**, but (there is evidence) that when we replace animal fats in our diets with seed oils we significantly increase the amount of harmful omega 6 fats in our cell membranes and this inevitably leads down a pathway to cancer and heart disease." Gillespie explains that seed oils didn't exist in our diet prior to 1920, and the industrial process used to extract oil from a seed is not natural.

And what is the reason behind this influx of vegetable and seed oils to replace fats such as butter and coconut oil? **The cost.** Gillespie argues it's much cheaper to produce (and for the consumer to buy) these oils in a factory than rear animals and slaughter them for their fat. He also proposes that essentially being animals ourselves, we produce animal fat, and the introduction of seed oils, especially when they oxidise, confuses our cell membranes, which can lead to conditions including heart disease.

In June 2014, *Time* magazine revisited the saturated fat debate. The front cover of the June 23 issue read, "Eat butter – Scientists labelled fat the enemy, why they were wrong". Referencing a meta-analysis in the *Annals of Internal Medicine, Time* concluded that "the removal of fats from our diet has led to an increase in consumption of carbohydrates and processed low-fat alternatives, which has contributed to record levels of diabetes and obesity.

We have been replacing real food with manmade, manufactured products that are created in a lab or a factory

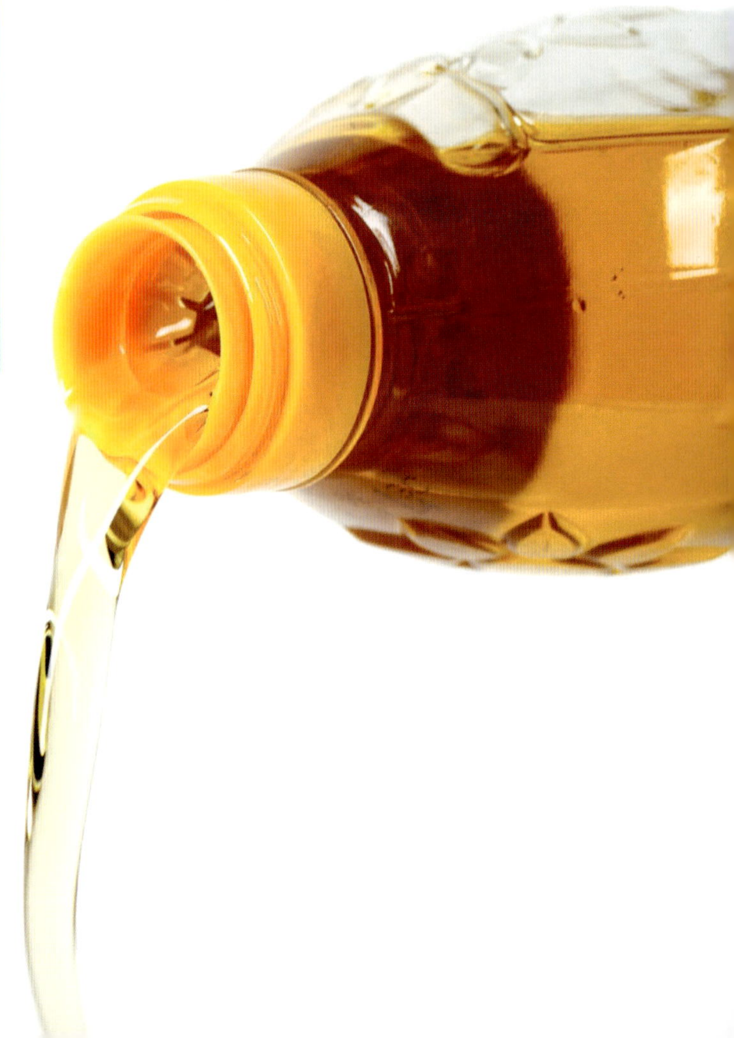

"When you consider that most low-fat or non-fat products are laden with salts, sugars and preservatives, continuing to seek out fat-free alternatives could be doing you more harm than good."

The **saturated fat debate continues**, whether organisations, including for diabetes and heart disease, will reverse their position on it in years to come is anyone's guess. What is important is that the debate exists, and that there is a plethora of information available for you to educate yourself and draw your own conclusions.

Just as an individual controls what they put on their plate each day, what medications they take under the advice of a medical professional, and what school of thinking they follow, the time will come when you will have to decide whether you continue to reduce or eliminate saturated fats or whether, as part of a balanced, wholefoods diet, you will consider reintroducing wholefoods that just happen to contain saturated fats.

The recipes in this book do contain saturated fats: animal fats in meat, butter, whole dairy and coconut milk and oil. The amounts used are not excessive.

Coconut oil has received a lot of negative press in recent years from those campaigning to reduce or eliminate saturated fats, but it has many benefits. It is more stable for cooking at higher temperatures than olive oil, and hasn't been treated in the same manner as vegetable or seed oils. It also tastes great and has a natural sweetness, meaning you don't need to add as much sweetener when using it in a dessert recipe. Coconut oil has medium chain saturated fatty acids, which are processed by the liver and converted to energy, as opposed to being directly stored as fat. Recent studies, including one by the Garvan Institute of Medical Research, have found that coconut oil can also **help improve insulin sensitivity**, and in turn is a great option for people with diabetes. Coconut oil can also boost immunity, aid in weight regulation, stabilise mood, and keep sugar cravings at bay.

Whether you choose to follow the recipes in this book to the letter, or substitute the full fat dairy and coconut oil for low-fat options is entirely **up to you**.

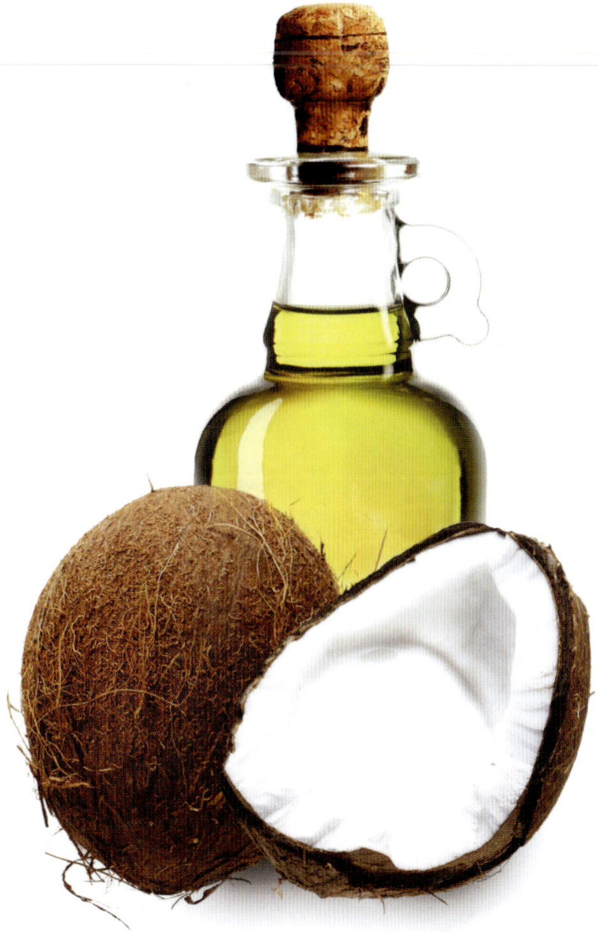

Recent studies have found that coconut oil can also help improve insulin sensitivity

The Low-Carb Question

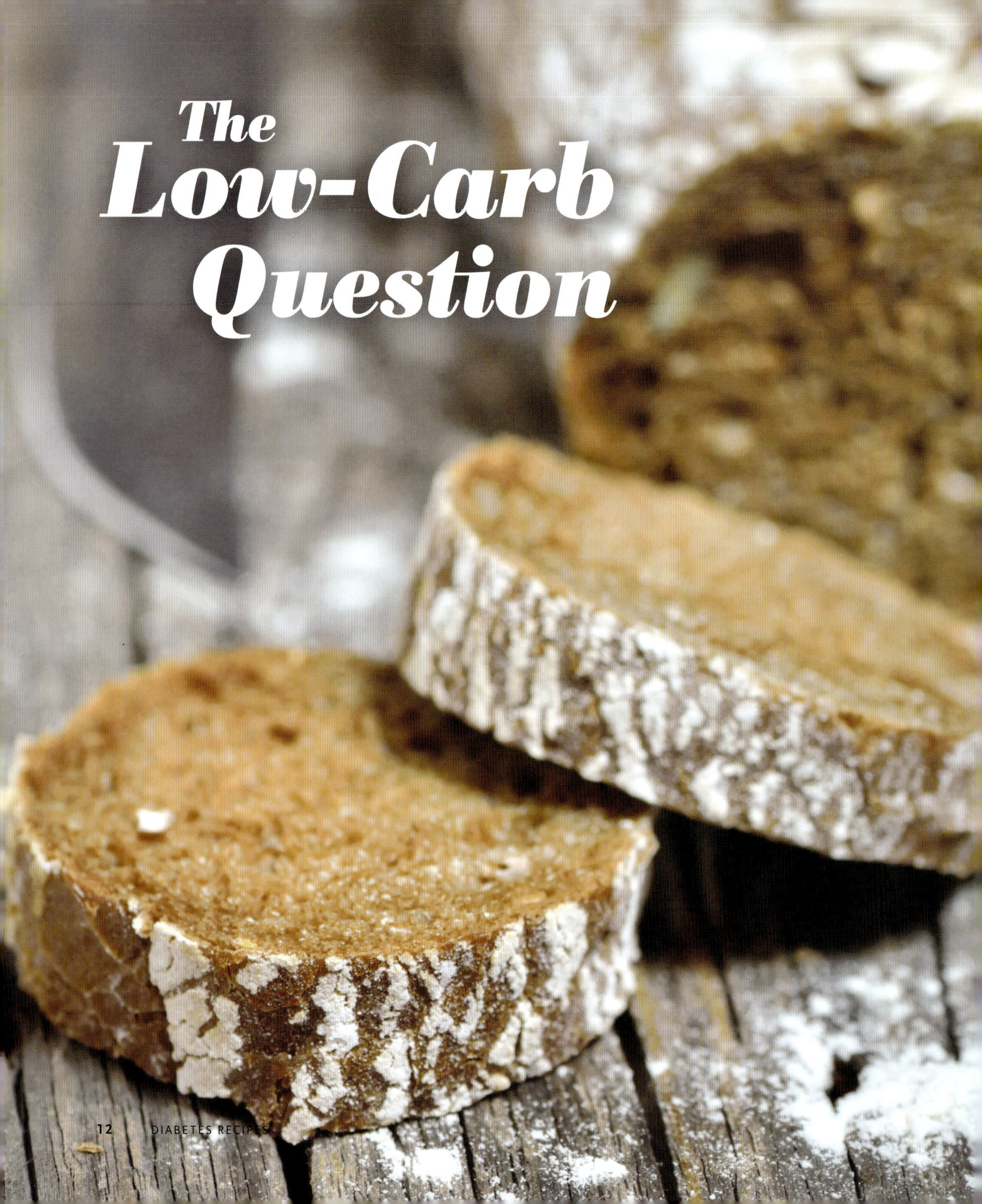

ALONG WITH promoting low-fat dairy and ditching saturated fats, diabetes organisations promote the consumption of a refined carbohydrate such as bread or pasta with every meal, something that could impact on your blood glucose levels. While there is nothing wrong with the occasional slice of toast for breakfast, dinner roll with your main course or treat such as a muffin, it's best to minimise starchy carbohydrates on a daily basis.

When a **carbohydrate is ingested** the body converts it into **glucose**, as it does with protein and fats. Just like protein and fats, not all carbohydrates are created equal, and consuming too many refined carbohydrates can result in blood glucose spikes. By monitoring your carbohydrate intake you can protect against the rise in blood sugar following meals. Beginning the day with a bowl of cereal and a slice of toast is a sure-fire way to jeopardise your blood glucose; although sometimes less convenient, it is a much better option to **eat a lean protein with good fats**, such as eggs with avocado, to help stabilise your blood sugar and set the course for the rest of the day.

In his book, *Wheat Belly*, William Davis MD addresses the dangers of wheat and grains in the diet, especially for a diabetic following mainstream medical advice. He reveals, "Two slices of whole wheat bread raise blood sugar higher than 6 teaspoons of sugar, higher than a Snickers bar."

By monitoring your carbohydrate intake you can protect against the rise in blood sugar following meals

In an interview discussing his book, Davis said he believes, "one of the most crucial aspects of the wheat conversation for people to understand is that the gliadin protein in wheat acts as an appetite-stimulant. People who consume the gliadin protein of wheat consume, on average, 400 more calories per day. People who eliminate the gliadin protein of wheat consume 400 calories less per day, even if calories, fat grams or portion sizes are unrestricted ... Put wheat flour, and thereby gliadin, into every product you can, you increase appetite, increase consumption, increase sales [for food companies]."

If the prospect of giving up your daily sandwich is overwhelming, begin **weaning yourself off refined carbohydrates** by making two days low-carb and focusing on increasing vegetable consumption to get the carbohydrates you need for fuel. Once you have conquered two days, why not try increasing to three or four days with a low-carb mindset? Avoid **starchy carbohydrates** including **white pasta and white bread** entirely. Create your meals around lean protein, as it can help stabilise blood sugar, and serve with a generous amount of non-starchy vegetables, including leafy greens.

As with any element of a diet, it is entirely dependent on the individual how far they take the low-carb train; some people may find their blood glucose levels are okay eating bread daily while others may experience frightening blood sugar spikes after one slice. It is best to **test how you react** to carbohydrates, even wholegrain breads and pastas, and determine what works best for you. No book, information pamphlet, organisation guidelines or medical advice can compare to how you feel and what your blood glucose does after eating a certain food, listen to your body.

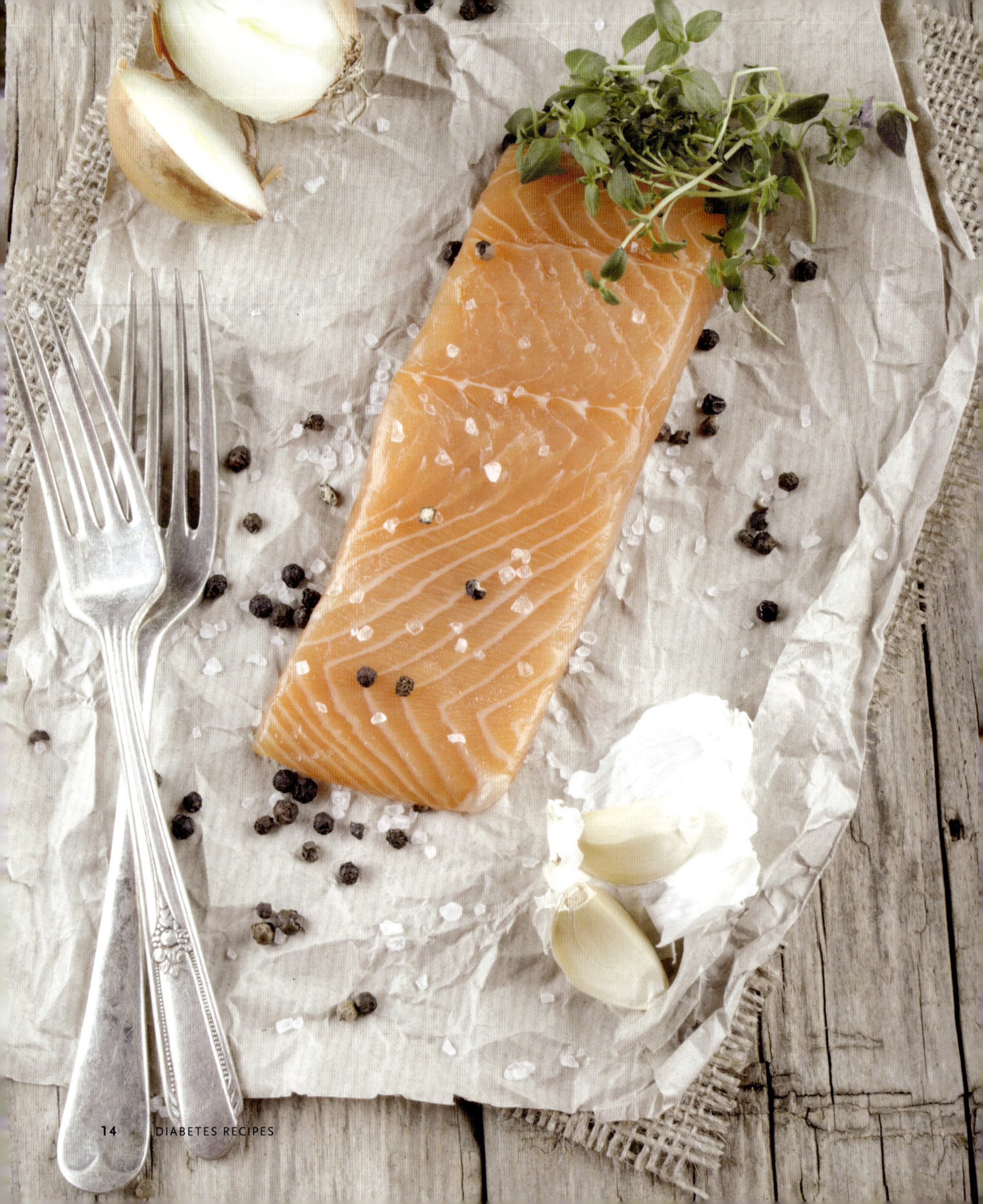

Diabetes, Heart Disease & Omega 3s

IF IT WASN'T troubling enough that you're now dealing with blood sugar levels spiking and dropping, we're also told by the American Diabetes Association that diabetics are twice as likely as non-diabetics to be struck down by heart disease, which can lead to heart attack or stroke.

The solution, they say, is to increase the amount of omega 3 fatty acids in your diet, both through increased consumption of fish, and through supplementation. Increased consumption of omega 3s is said to be beneficial for supporting cell health and helping with blood clotting. It's also said to be valuable in improving insulin sensitivity and is recommended for pre-diabetics to ward off a full diagnosis of diabetes.

Omega 3s are considered "essential" fatty acids because our bodies cannot produce them and we need to source them from our food supply. When we cannot consume adequate amounts of omega 3s through our food we are advised to turn to supplements, such as fish oil or krill oil, to boost our intake. Not surprisingly, as with most things concerning our health these days, there is debate surrounding the effectiveness of these supplements, with the National Institute for Health and Care Excellence suggesting the effect of fish oil supplements "could be minimal"; their study is backed up by several including one by the New England Journal of Medicine.

Whether you choose to follow mainstream medical advice or embark on your own research into the divided opinion, it seems the best approach to making sure you meet your omega 3 needs is caution.

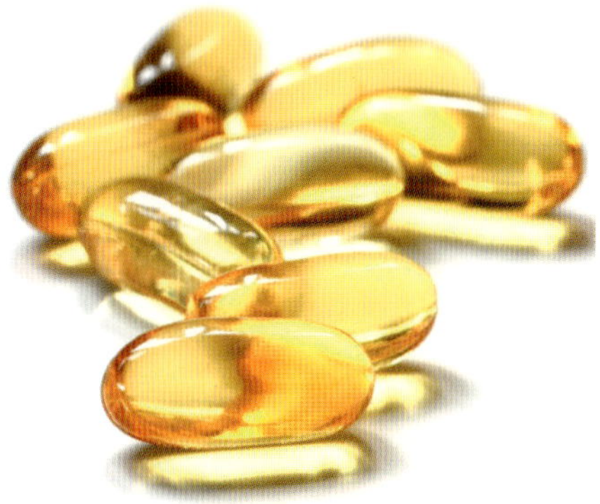

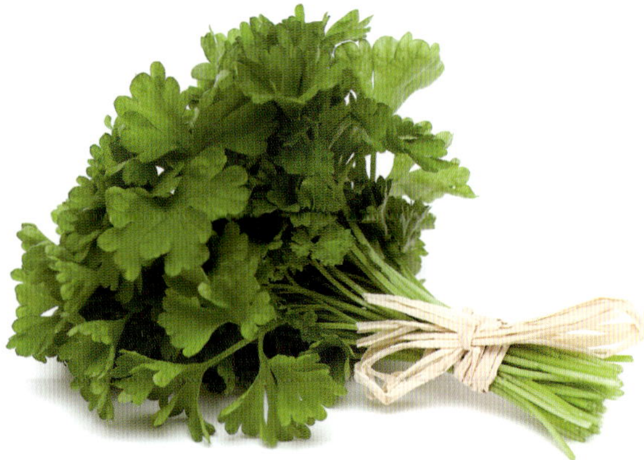

When purchasing fresh fish, make sure you buy from a trusted source, the same as you would when seeking organic produce. Go for **wild caught fish** as opposed to farmed fish, especially when buying **Atlantic Salmon**. Farmed salmon can contain high levels of antibiotics, used to treat parasites, and high levels of Polychlorinated Biphenyl toxins (**PCBs**). PCBs are part of a group of toxic and harmful persistent organic pollutants (POPs) produced in the 1970s that then leached into waterways and sewerage systems. They were mainly used in coolants and lubricants for electrical equipment but could also be found in paint and dye amongst other things. Despite being banned in the late 1970s by countries such as the United States of America and Australia, PCBs remain in the environment and can be carried by animals, such as fish.

There are also many fish listed as threatened species that boast **potentially high levels of mercury and PCBs**, including Bluefin tuna and Orange Roughy. The Environmental Defense Fund (EDF) recommends steering clear of these species, in addition to the farmed salmon. Aim for mackerel, barramundi, oysters, mussels, sardines, trout and sustainable tuna if choosing seafood as an omega 3 source.

Fish is a great source of **healthy protein** and should not be omitted if you enjoy the taste and can reap its many nutritional benefits without exposing yourself to its potential health risks. There are many other great sources of omega 3s you can include in your diet such as walnuts, flaxseeds, pumpkin seeds, Brussels sprouts, cauliflower, eggs, grass-fed beef, kale, spinach and parsley.

Go for wild caught fish as opposed to farmed fish, especially when buying Atlantic Salmon

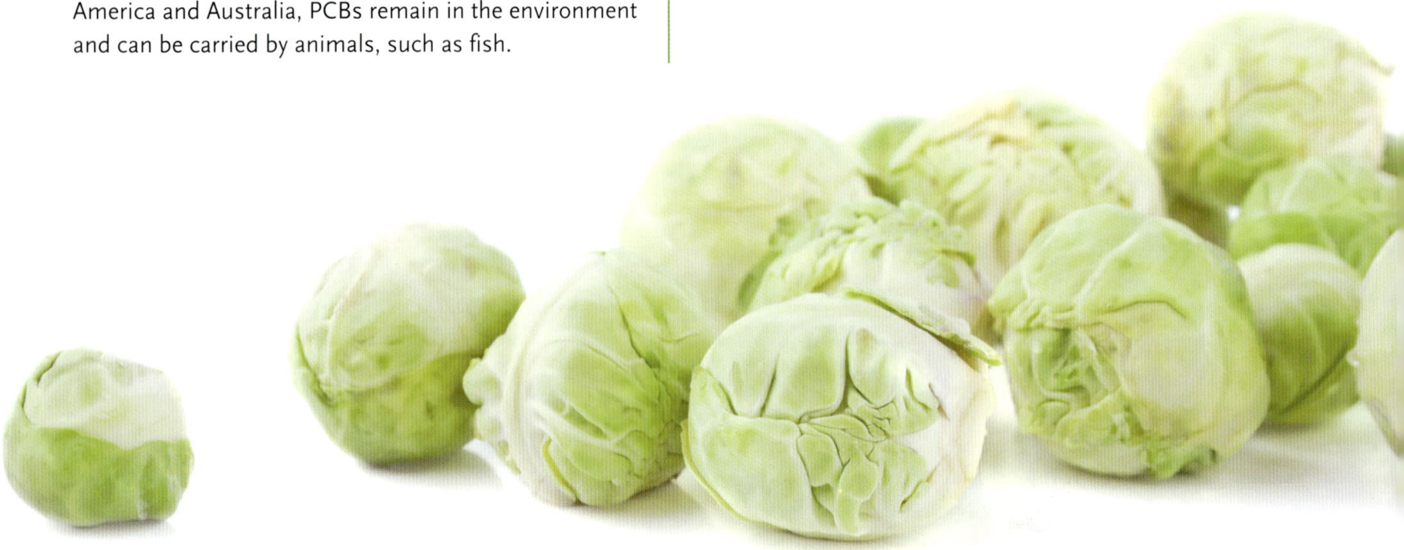

Low Sugar Living

THE LATEST guideline promoted by official diabetes associations is that sugar no longer needs to be avoided like the plague by diabetics. Don't start celebrating just yet; put down that block of chocolate!

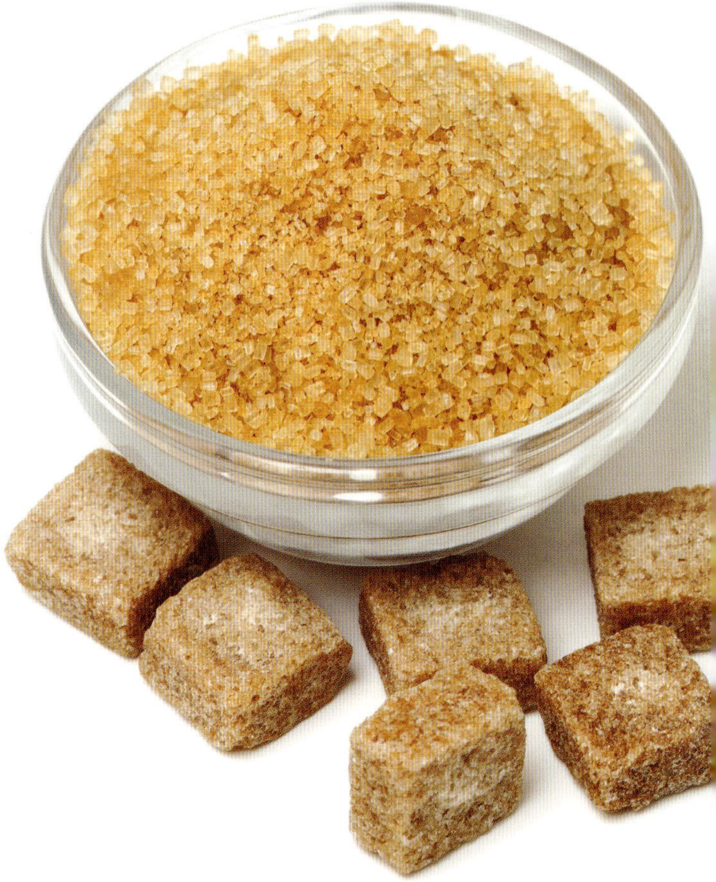

There are **some foods with natural sugars** that should be added to your shopping list every week. They're not hard to find in a supermarket because there's an entire section devoted to them and they have no nutrition labels to try and decode. Of course I'm talking about fruits and vegetables.

The fructose that occurs naturally in fruits and vegetables comes wrapped in fibre and with the added bonus of a variety of minerals and nutrients. Our bodies are designed to process the unrefined fructose in **two pieces of fruit daily**, with the fibre helping to slow the absorption of the sugar into our body.

The problem with sugar consumption occurs when it is added to other foods. Consider your fellow shopper's trolley next time you are in the supermarket: how much of its contents are fresh produce and how much is packaged and processed foods? When you increase the amount of pre-made food you consume, products that were manufactured in factories and have had preservatives added to extend the shelf life, you automatically increase your sugar, and often salt, consumption. Taking the time to **read a nutrition label** will highlight this to you if you weren't already aware.

Since sugar rations were abolished following the end of the Second World War, **food manufacturers** have been adding it to anything and everything. Sauces, dressings, pre-marinated meat, muesli bars, low-fat products, cereal, bread, yoghurt, the list goes on. We've become addicted to the sweet taste of sugar and it's time to reduce its impact in your life by getting back to basics and preparing meals from scratch.

Healthy eating shopping tips

1. STICK TO THE PERIMETER OF THE STORE. Here you'll find the freshest food, from produce to meat and dairy. Of course this rule can bend somewhat, you'll have to venture down the aisles for spices, oil, toilet paper etc. They say two-thirds of your dinner plate should be **plant based**, and the same applies to your shopping trolley. If your local supermarket lacks variety or quality when it comes to fruits and vegetables, seek out your nearest speciality produce store and stock up!

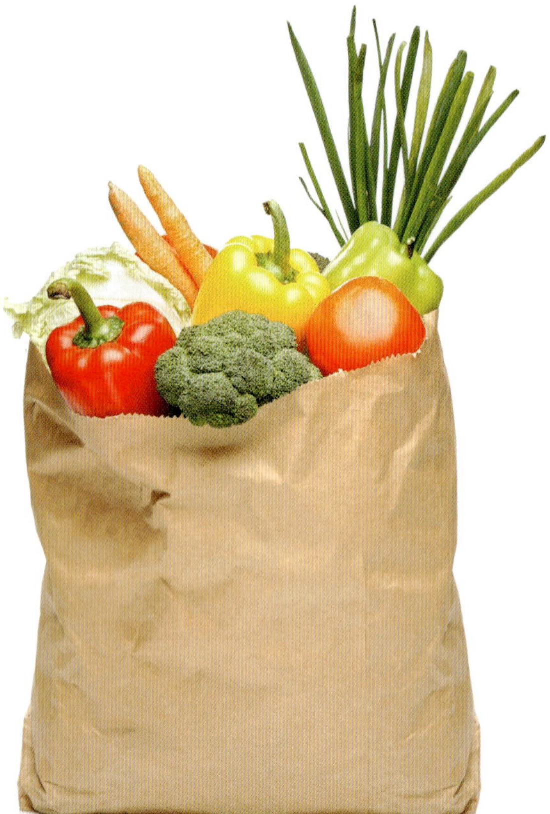

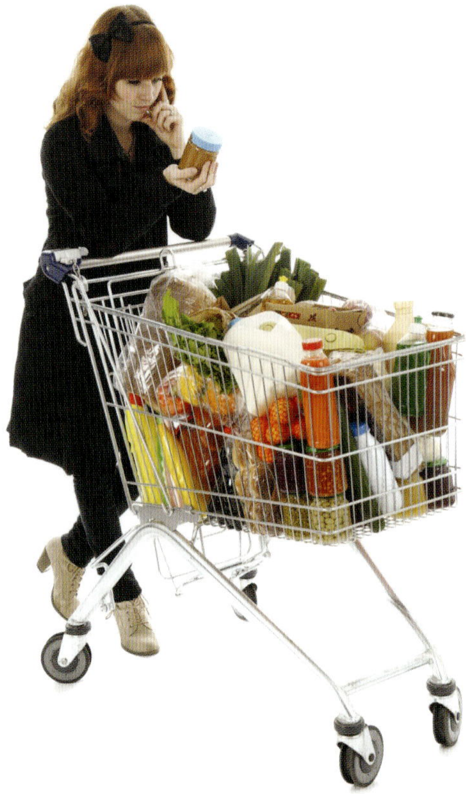

2. READ LABELS. Another no-brainer but for many a trip to the supermarket is quick-in and quick-out, grab the essentials, be tempted by a special, and zip through the self checkout. Slow down. Take the time to read the label. What are the ingredients? Do you understand what they all are? Can you pronounce them even? How much sugar and salt is in the product? Is there a better option? **Serving sizes** can be deceiving so it's always best to base your decision on the 'Per 100g' column, which also makes it easier to work out the percentage of sodium, carbohydrates etc. Ingredients must be listed in **descending weight order** so if sugar appears first, immediately drop the packet and run.

3. DEDICATE TIME FOR FOOD SHOPPING. If you're in a rush, you're more likely to grab what's close or on special. Set aside an hour one week to go to the supermarket alone or with your shopping partner and walk the aisles reading and comparing labels. Pick up the brands and items you would usually buy and read the package, compare with competing brands and see if another product is a better choice. Once you've dedicated a shopping trip to this it will reduce the overall time of subsequent trips as you'll know which products to add to your trolley and which to skip completely.

4. PLAN AHEAD. Write a shopping list and **stick to it!** Put your invisible blinkers on and know where you have to go; avoid wandering the aisles and letting yourself be tempted by things you don't need. If it helps, plan the coming week's meals and snacks on the weekend and write your list according to what you'll need. Be firm. Do not deviate from the list and no matter how tempting something looks, be strong.

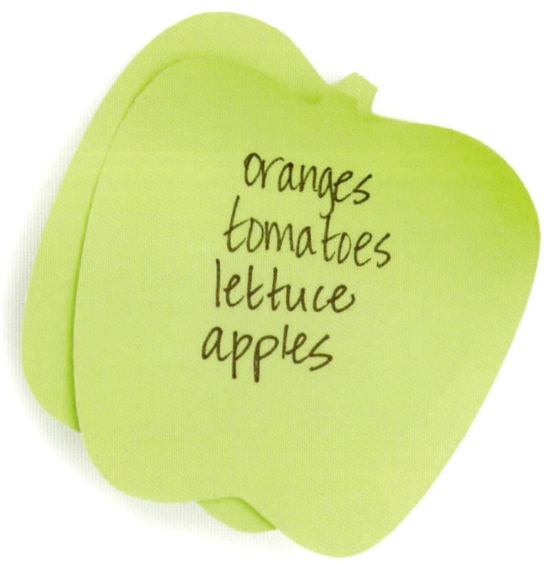

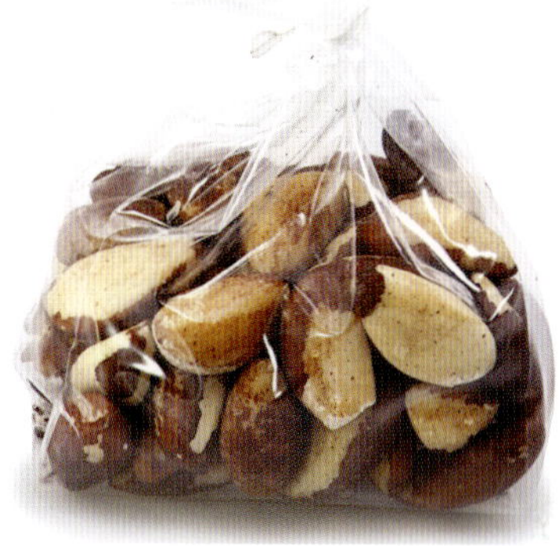

5. DON'T SHOP HUNGRY. It's an age-old rule that makes a lot of sense. If you go to the store on an empty stomach you'll likely come home with bags full of stuff you really shouldn't be eating. Biscuits, ice cream, chips, convenience meals, they all look tempting when our stomach starts to grumble. Worst case scenario; buy a **small bag of nuts** when you begin your shopping to nibble on as you make your way through the supermarket.

6. RESIST THE IMPULSE BUY AND AVOID FRONT OF STORE AND END OF AISLE DISPLAYS. Huge displays adorn the entryways to most supermarkets and the ends of aisles, advertising the latest competition or presenting a towering display of a super special that's such a great deal you'd be crazy not to put two of each flavour into your trolley immediately. Their goal is obvious, catch you unawares and make you seize on the **impulse buy**. Occasionally the produce department specials will seep into this area, and you might be lucky to snag yourself a fresh bargain or a close-to-use-by-date special, but more often than not we're talking slabs of soft drink and towers of boxed biscuits and chips. Stick to your plan, stick to your list, and resist the impulse buy!

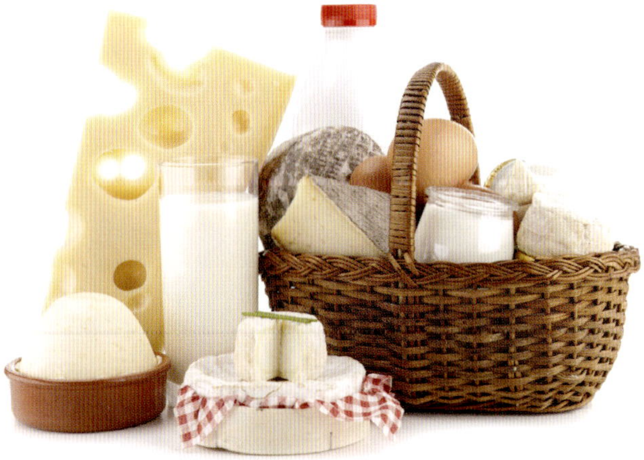

7. AVOID ANYTHING LABELLED LITE, LOW-FAT OR FAT FREE. Fat isn't necessarily a bad thing, our brains actually need it to thrive and it satiates our hunger. The reason to avoid foods labelled Lite, Low-fat or Fat free is that when fat is taken out of a food, sugar or other substitutes (including milk powder or salt) are usually put in. The product still has to taste good enough to sell (and eat), right? Go full fat dairy; butter, milk, yoghurt and cheese. Not convinced? Rule #2 – read and compare the labels! Remember, it's better to consume smaller amounts of a **natural food** made with minimal human interference than go to town on "food" concocted in laboratories and factories. Butter from grass fed cows will always trump mass produced margarine made from vegetable oil when it comes to health benefits.

8. AVOID PRODUCTS WITH MORE THAN 5 INGREDIENTS. There are many reasons why we reach for a bottle of premade sauce, a sachet of flavouring to add to a casserole, or an entire meal frozen in a cardboard box. Laziness and lack of time rank highly on the list as we move further away from home cooked meals to home prepared meals. No one is suggesting you need to grow your own tomatoes, harvest and process them into your own tomato sauce and paste, but a basic pasta sauce has less than 5 ingredients; it's a good rule of thumb to keep in mind when perusing the supermarket shelves.

9. BRING THE KIDS ALONG. Controversial, I know. Many will suggest leaving the kids at home when doing the food shopping to avoid the "inevitable" temper tantrum in the cereal or biscuit aisle, and sometimes this is the best plan of attack. For the other times, treat your children with the intelligence they have and deserve, and discuss what you're buying, and not buying, with them. If you begin educating them about food choices and the power of advertising from a young age, you may be surprised how well it sticks.

10. TREAT YOURSELF. Don't forget that a treat now and then goes a long way.

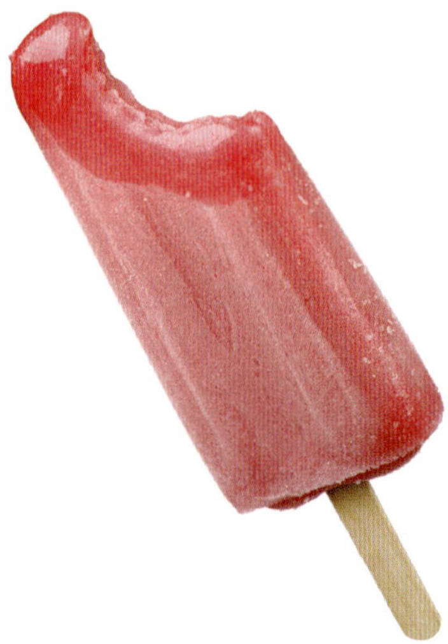

Sweeteners

RAW HONEY

Raw honey, that is locally sourced and hasn't been heat-treated, has an abundance of healing properties to consider. You won't find this type of honey on your supermarket shelf, anything sitting there has been heat treated and processed to remove all of the beneficial elements and leave only the sweetness. Your local farmers' market is a great source for raw honey, as is the Internet. It's amazing what you can source online these days; with many metropolitan areas boasting rooftop honey schemes ensuring local bees and minimal human interference. Raw honey ensures a premium product that has retained most or all of the beneficial enzymes, natural vitamins and antioxidants. It is anti viral, anti bacterial, promotes good digestive health and can be a powerful aid in treating allergies, particularly hay fever. A little bit goes a long way so you'll find a jar of raw honey can keep you going for many months, if not longer. If you can't source good quality raw honey don't substitute with a supermarket shelf brand, simply avoid it entirely.

MAPLE SYRUP

As with honey, maple syrup comes in myriad of qualities and the more you pay, the purer the product will be. It is incredibly sweet so only a small amount goes a long way in recipes; I'm not suggesting dousing a stack of pancakes in the stuff, as it is traditionally used for. Its health benefits include a high level of manganese, which is great for energy and in strengthening your immunity, and high levels of zinc, also good for the immune system and for reproductive health. Look for organic Grade A pure maple syrup and avoid maple "flavoured" syrup, which is a highly refined product lacking the benefits of the pure product.

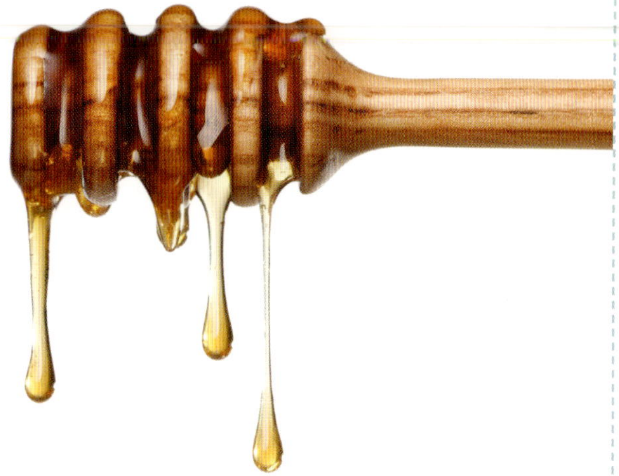

RICE MALT SYRUP

Rice malt syrup is fructose free and is made from brown rice using a process where the rice is cultured with enzymes to break down the starch; it's then cooked until it becomes a syrup. Rice malt syrup is a complex carbohydrate with maltose (malt sugar) and a small amount of glucose. It can usually be found in the health food aisle of most supermarkets, in health stores or online. It is relatively cheap and a little tends to go a long way. Rice malt syrup is a great option because of its low cost, ease of use and taste but it should still be used in moderation and not become an everyday product. When buying, look for a brand with 100% rice in the ingredients list.

MEDJOOL DATES

On the whole, dates and other dried fruits should be consumed sparingly. The dehydration process concentrates the fruit's natural fructose as water is removed and the fruit shrinks in size, often meaning you end up eating a larger quantity. However, when used in desserts or sweet treats sparingly, especially when shared with friends and family, including dates boasts some health benefits in addition to their great taste. They are high in magnesium and zinc, and full of fibre, just remember to consume them in moderation. I opt for Medjool dates over other varieties as they are softer and blend much better.

Ditch the drinks

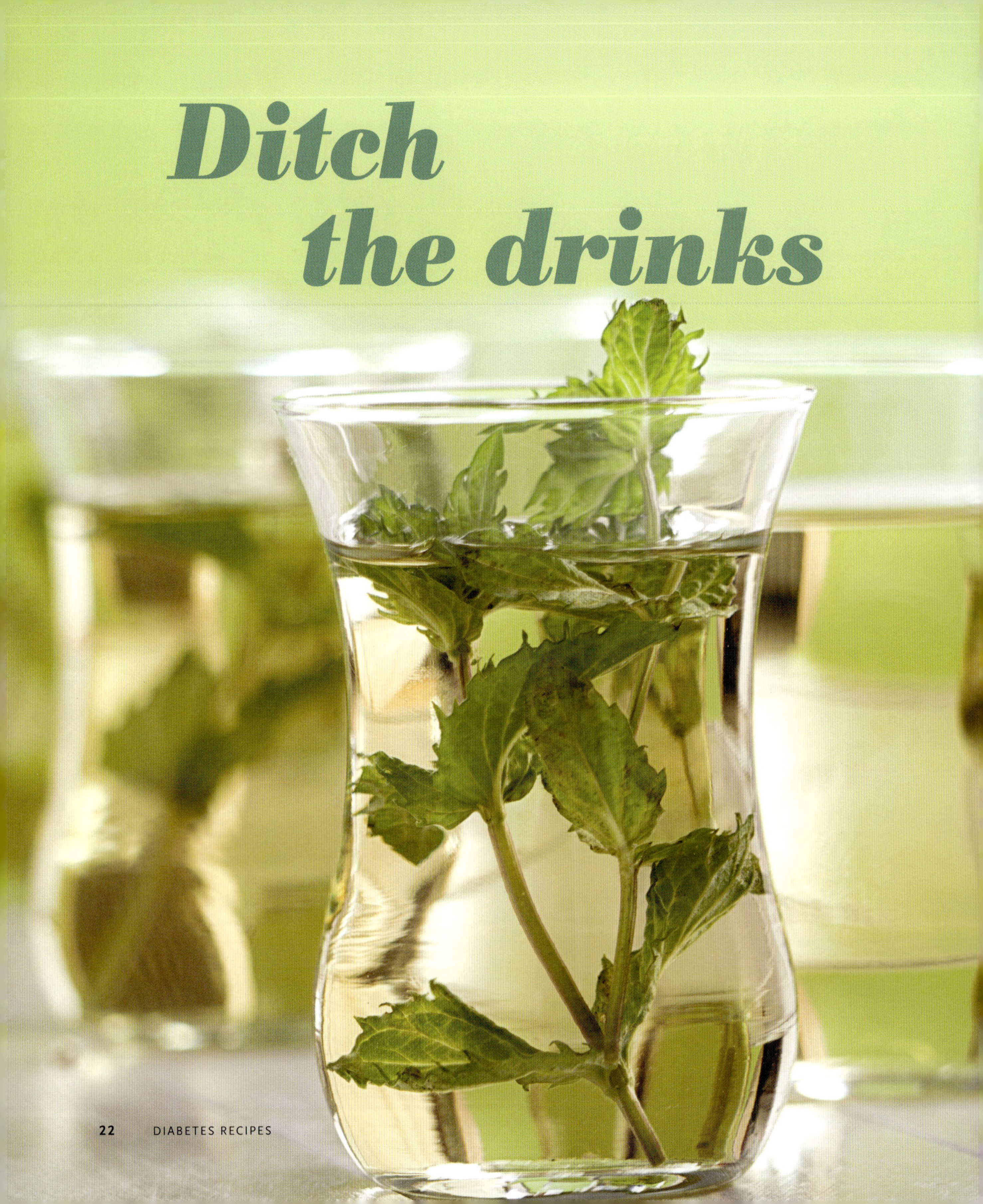

THERE IS ONLY one liquid we need to survive and that is water. Every other beverage that we consume has been introduced into our diet for pleasure. Our diets are now ruled by pleasure over purpose, and while it is nice to have the occasional sweetened drink, it should never be a daily occurrence, especially for people with diabetes.

Immediately eliminate **soft drinks, sodas, cordials** and **fruit juices** from your diet. These liquid sugar cocktails will only send your blood glucose levels into a frenzy and overwork your liver.

Fruit juice has long been masquerading as a healthy alternative to soft drinks but it is packed with **excess fructose** that your body cannot process in large quantities. If you're craving fruit juice try **diluting it with water** or making your own juice at home and sticking to the 80-20 rule: 80% vegetables and 20% fruit. You'll find that you only need half an apple to sweeten a juice once you reset your body and taste buds to appreciate the natural sweetness in real food.

Drinking **herbal teas** throughout the day is a great way to keep hydrated, and can easily be turned into iced teas for a refreshing drink on a hot day. Boost the flavour of your tea by adding citrus peel, fresh herbs or slices of fresh fruit when it is brewing.

Reset your body and taste buds to appreciate the natural sweetness in real food

Alcohol should be **limited** but does not need to be eliminated when managing your diabetes. Stick to **red wine, beer** or **straight spirits** to limit blood sugar spikes. Champagne and white wines are fine to have occasionally, but mixed drinks with sugary bases should be avoided.

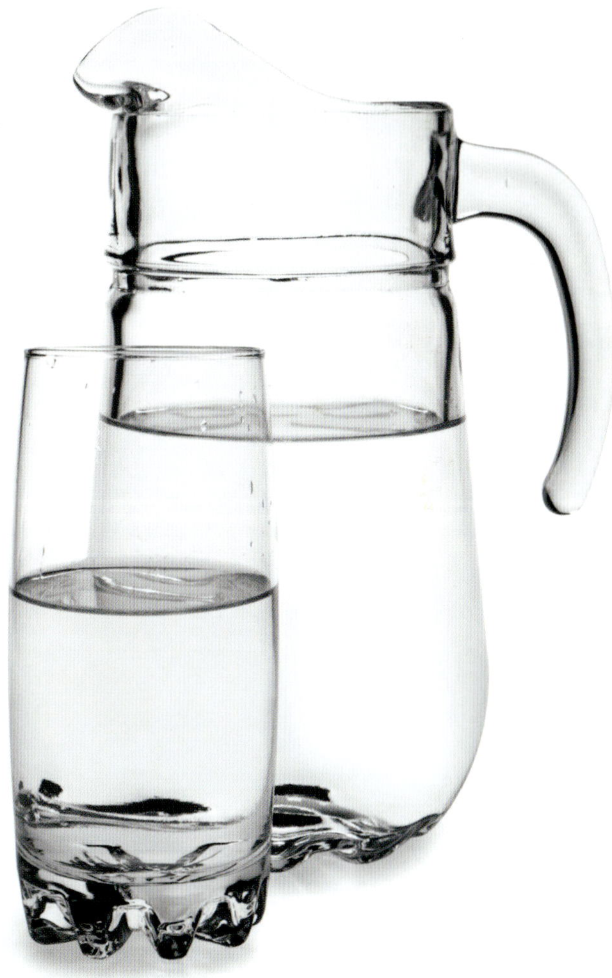

Does Size Matter?

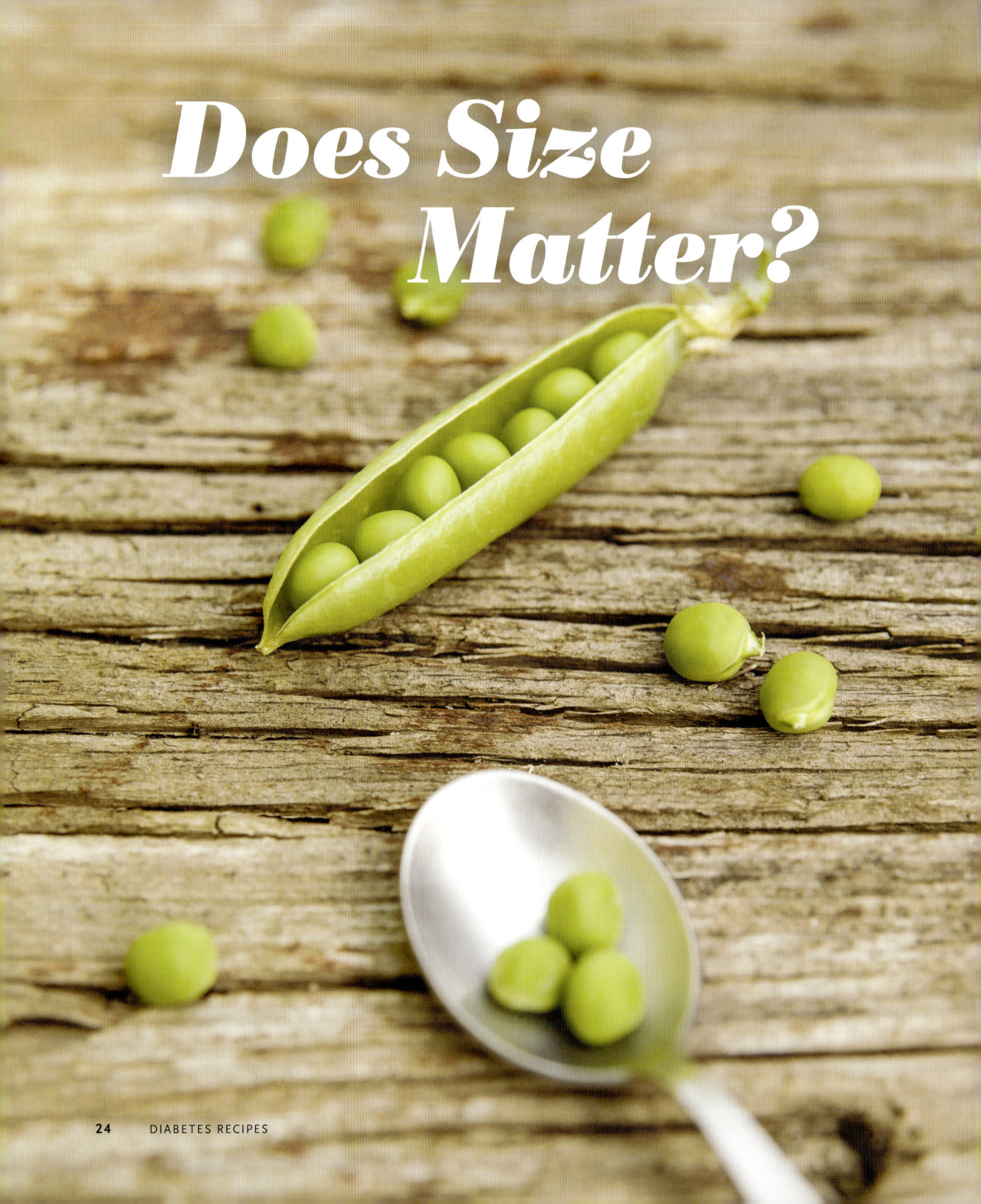

IT'S NOT JUST the type of food you eat but also the amount of it that can impact on your blood glucose levels and control. Does size matter? Absolutely.

Being **aware of portion sizes** can not only save you from blood glucose spikes, but will also make it easier to **maintain a healthy weight**, helping to reduce the likelihood of diabetes complications. People with diabetes commonly feel hungry directly after eating a meal because their blood glucose levels rise quickly and then fall. The **larger the meal** you eat the more likely these blood sugar spikes are, and so the theory goes that by sticking to smaller portion sizes your blood glucose is less likely to spike and crash.

Many organisations encourage **measuring** or **weighing your food** to control portions, or following the suggested serving size on a nutritional label. Measuring or weighing food is not always practical, can reduce your overall enjoyment of the meal you are about to eat, and can be hard to maintain when eating out, socialising with friends or while on holidays.

Following a nutritional label can be handy when enjoying an occasional snack, but if you are looking at a nutritional label then you are holding a packaged and most likely processed food. **Portion control** is important and can help you lose or maintain weight as well as stabilise blood glucose, but the same can be said for eliminating processed foods and increasing servings of fresh, whole foods, as well as cooking from scratch. It's also important to remember that serving sizes on nutritional labels are **dictated by your country's dietary guidelines**, and often follow the food pyramid system that advises low-fat dairy and equal weighting with vegetables, cereals, grains and carbohydrates.

You should be conscious of everything you eat, but by eliminating refined and starchy carbohydrates and sugar, and reducing wholegrain carbohydrates with every meal, such as bread, counting calories becomes less important. By choosing quality protein, nutrient-dense, non-starchy vegetables, and a small amount of good fats such as avocado, your body can naturally stop you from overeating.

A diet high in refined sugar and carbohydrates will contribute to a person's inability to control the amount of food they eat. By **reducing the amount of excess fructose** and **starchy carbohydrates** in your diet, you release the body's natural ability to **regulate appetite**. You may have often asked yourself why a steak or even cheese and crackers fills you up faster than a packet of cookies or a bowl of ice cream. Your three appetite hormones, insulin, leptin and cholecystokinin don't respond to the flood of fructose that enters the body when you eat a sugary food, and so you feel like you can eat more and more without filling up. Meanwhile your blood sugar levels are going crazy and you're still left hungry. Once you reduce your intake of excess refined sugar and refined carbohydrates such as bread and pasta, you should find yourself **more aware of when you are truly hungry** as well as finding you feel full from eating less food.

It may take some time to recalibrate your system if your day usually starts off with cereal and bread, or if your sweet tooth has persisted despite your diabetes diagnosis, but given time you can **reset your mind and your taste buds** to think and eat the right sized portions of fresh and whole foods.

By choosing quality protein, nutrient-dense, non-starchy vegetables, and a small amount of good fats such as avocado, your body can naturally stop you from overeating

Portion control tips

Don't skip meals and you'll be less likely to overeat. Start the day by skipping breakfast and you greatly increase the likelihood of overindulging in a mid-morning snack or eating a larger lunch than usual. Skip lunch and you might find yourself craving starchy carbohydrates by dinner or raiding the cupboard for a sweet treat after dinner.

Don't follow the suggested "serving size" on a nutritional label. Packaged foods should not be an everyday item. Avoid packaged biscuits, crackers, pretzels, chips, muesli and snack bars. Snack on small pieces of fruit, vegetable sticks, homemade dip such as hummus or guacamole, or a finger-sized serving of cheese such as haloumi.

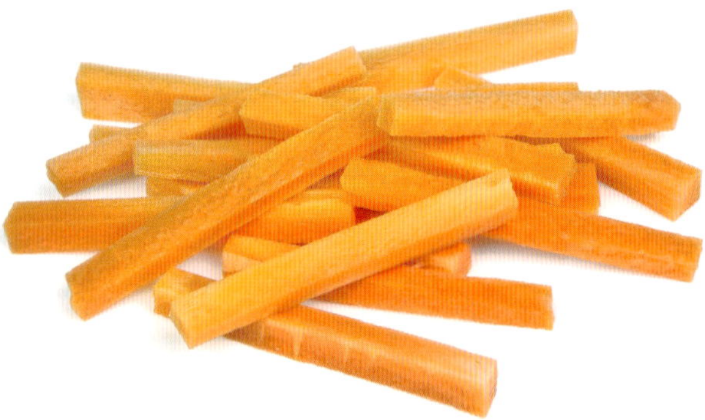

Divide your plate for optimal portion control. Ensure your plate is half vegetables, ¼ protein and ¼ good fats or unrefined carbohydrates.

Eat the bulk of the vegetables on your plate first followed by the protein to fill up before eating any carbohydrates such as rice, pasta or bread.

Aim to go **no longer than 5 waking hours without eating**, whether a main meal or a protein-rich snack.

Avoid eating or snacking while **watching television**, you'll likely be distracted and eat more than you should.

If wanting a treat at the cinema, resist the upgrade to a large combo and stick to a small popcorn and bottle of water. Better yet, make your own **healthier popcorn** or snacks at home and smuggle them in.

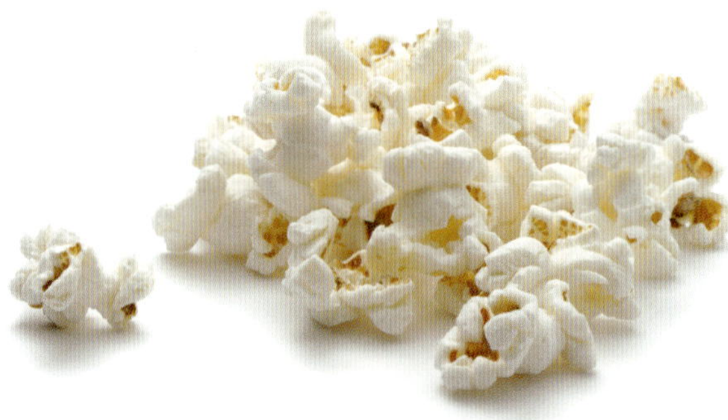

When choosing the **portion size of meat**, aim for a piece no larger than the size of your palm or a deck of cards. If choosing to eat cereal, eat no more than 1 cup's worth or a serving about the size of your fist.

Switch **dinner plates** with side or salad plates to reduce the amount of food in front of you.

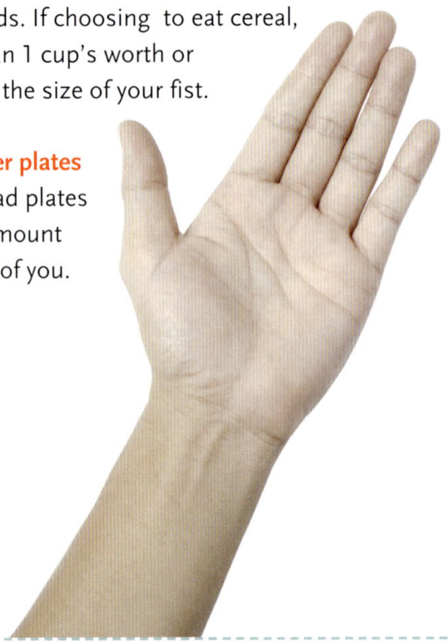

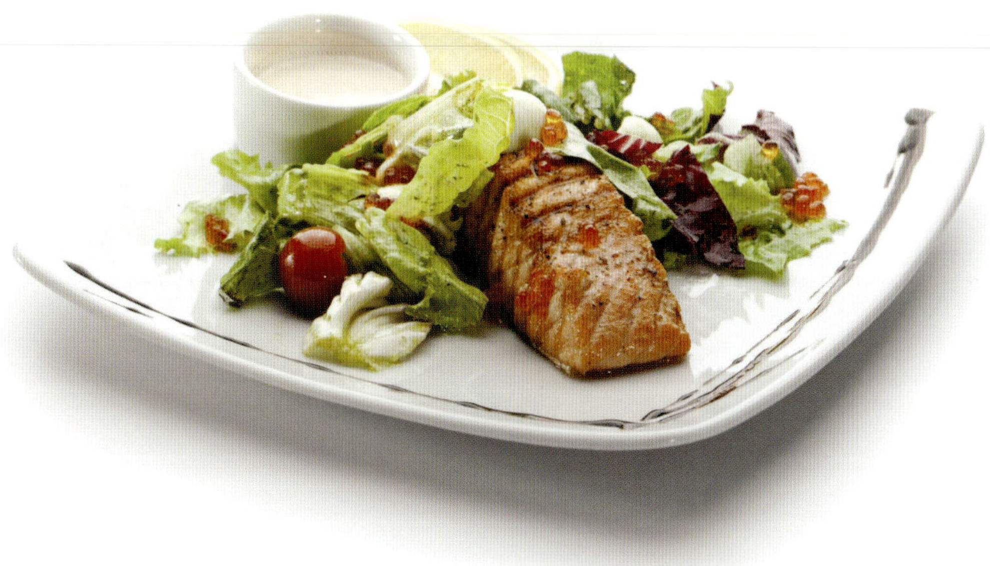

- **Remember restaurants usually serve larger meal sizes, choose to split a large main with someone** rather than eat it all yourself or waste food, or ask for any leftovers to be boxed up for you to take home. Alternatively, order an entree and a side rather than one main course.

- **Avoid buffet restaurants** and the temptation to eat more food and get your "money's worth".

- **Avoid second helpings** directly after eating. Wait 10 – 15 minutes after eating your first serve to see if you are really hungry before filling your plate up again.

- If you're full, **don't force yourself to eat everything on the plate.** Transfer leftovers to a container and store in the refrigerator for the next day rather than overeating to clean your plate.

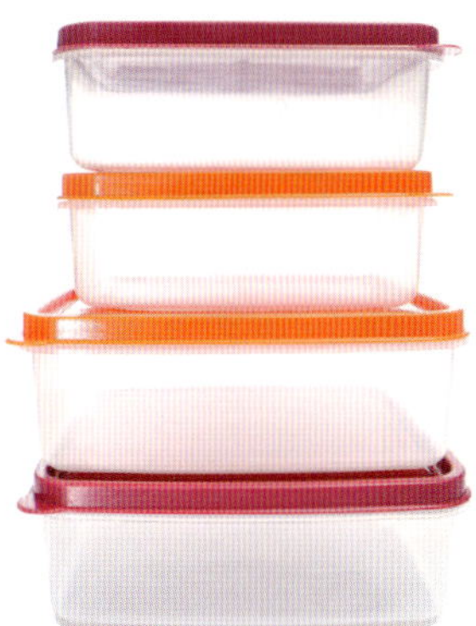

- **Choose smaller pieces of fruit** when food shopping rather than large ones. If you have a large piece of fruit, consider cutting it in half and eating one portion in the morning and one in the afternoon. Aim to eat more vegetables than fruit and include a variety of vegetables, especially leafy greens.

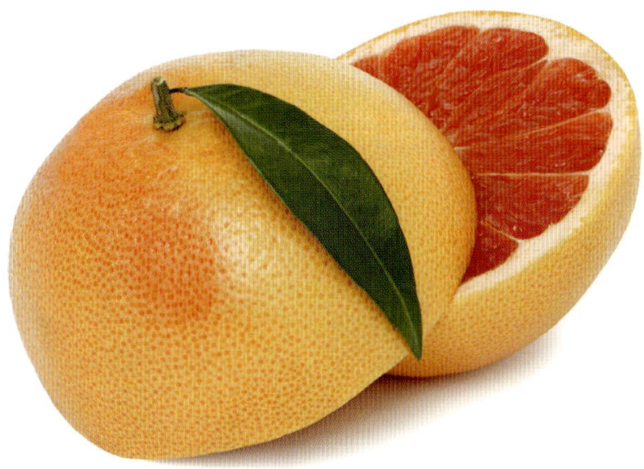

- If you have any **emotional eating issues** that may lead to binging or overeating less than ideal foods, deal with them by talking to a trained professional or trusted friend.

Top Foods to Stabilise Blood Sugar

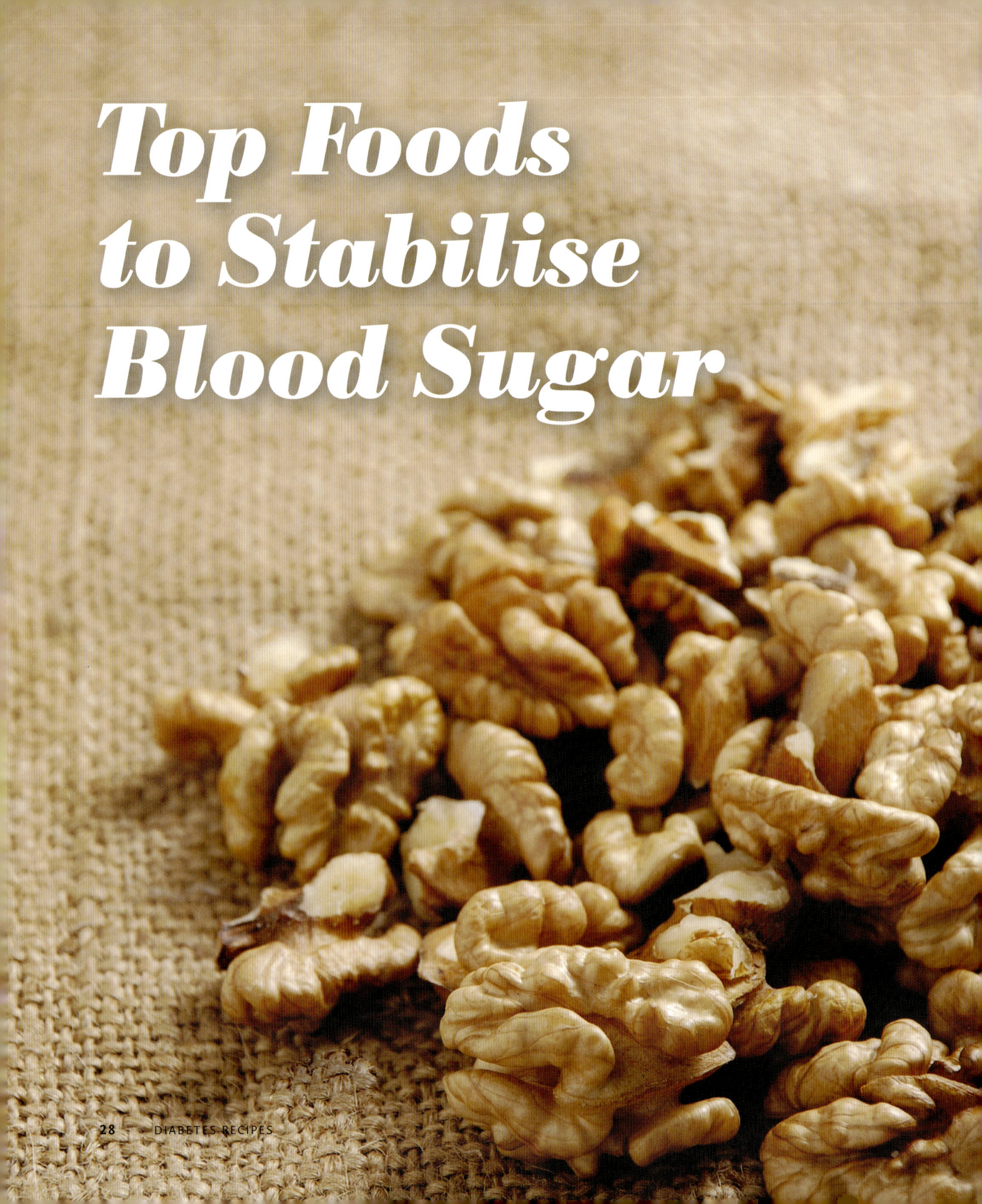

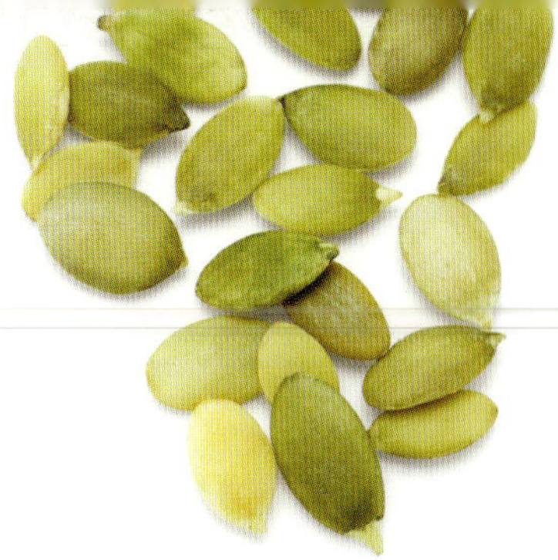

RAW NUTS & SEEDS: Nuts such as walnuts, Brazil nuts, macadamia nuts and pine nuts, and seeds including pumpkin (pepitas), sesame and sunflower are nutrient dense and bite-sized, making them perfect as a snack or added into meals. Nuts and seeds provide slow burning fuel for your body, which can help in regulating blood sugar levels between meals.

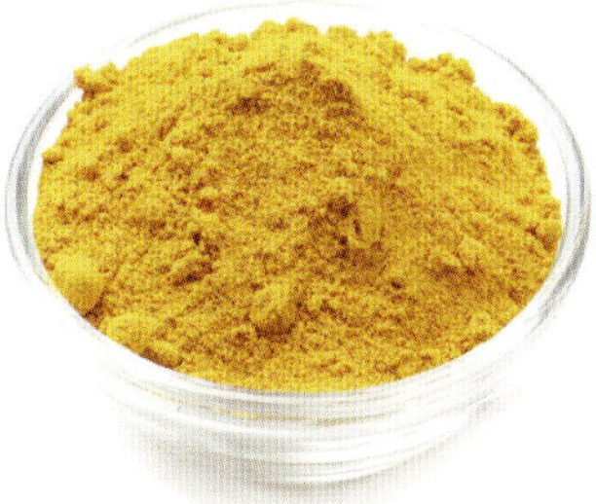

SPICES: Cinnamon and turmeric top the list of spices that help stabilise blood sugar while also adding flavour to a simple breakfast dish or a delicious curry for dinner. Cinnamon contains polyphenol, which helps your body lower its blood sugar levels in a similar way to how insulin works.

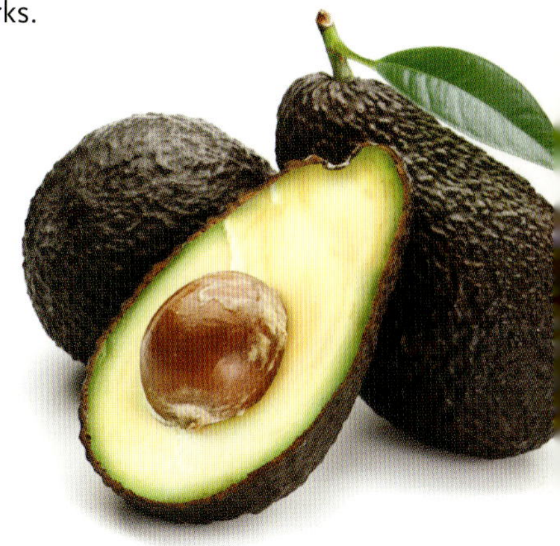

AVOCADO: The wonder fruit is loved for its creamy texture and nutty taste. It's great eaten as a snack, added to salads or even whipped up into a tasty dessert. Avocadoes contain more soluble fibre than any other fruit, helping stabilise blood glucose levels. When added to a carbohydrate-rich meal, such as a sandwich made with bread, avocadoes can help slow down the speed of digestion. The monounsaturated fat found in avocadoes, the same as found in olive oil, will keep you feeling fuller longer, helping you avoid snacking and spiking blood sugar levels.

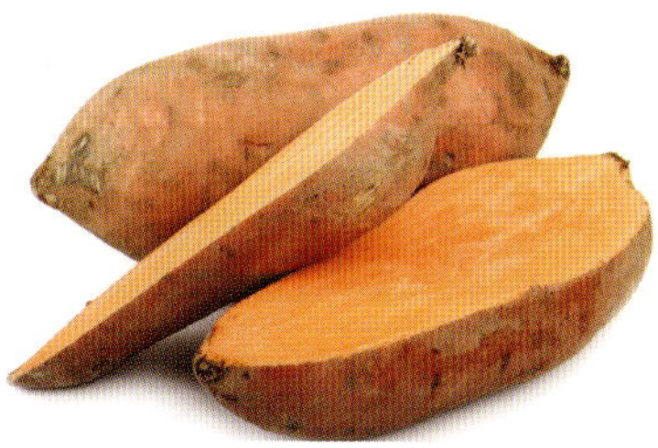

SWEET POTATO: The much-healthier cousin to the common white potato, this vegetable is just as versatile in creating delicious mashes and crispy oven baked chips without sending your blood sugar on a rollercoaster ride. Packed with beta-carotene and soluble fibre, this winning combination helps your body regulate insulin and blood glucose levels.

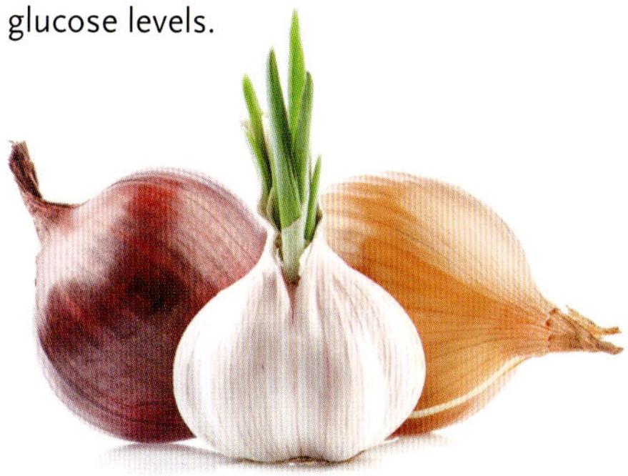

GARLIC & ONIONS: A great combination in any meal, individually both ingredients help stabilise blood sugar and boast high antioxidant properties. Garlic is best eaten raw to maximise its benefits.

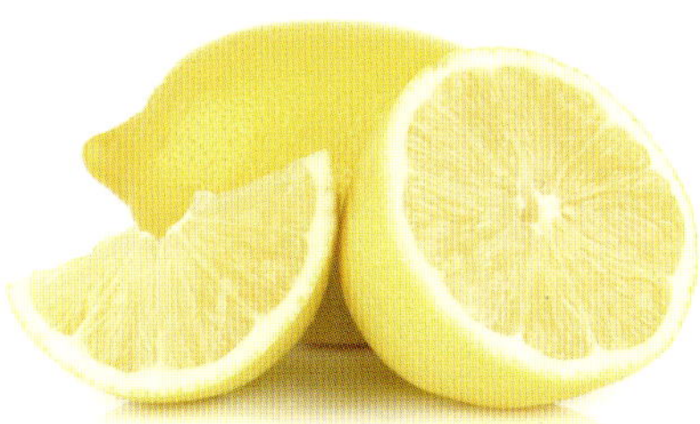

LEMONS & CITRUS: Further to its blood glucose lowering abilities, the acidity level of lemons can help reduce the overall glucose index (GI) of a meal.

Stress & Diabetes:

A Match Made in Heaven

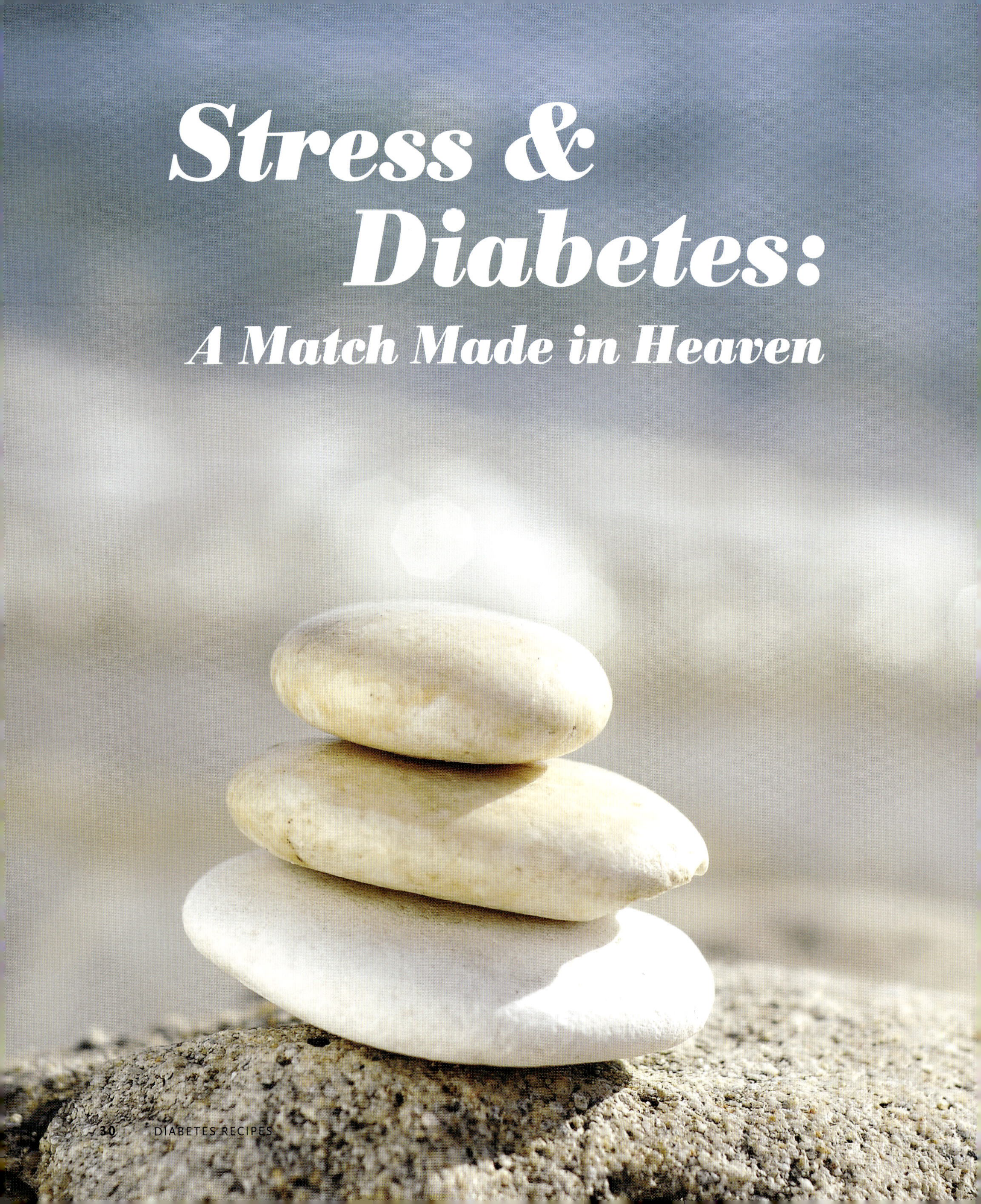

THERE'S ONE THING that will continue to derail your management of diabetes even when taking medication and maintaining a balanced diet: stress.

When you **experience stress**, whether emotional or physical, your body releases a **stress hormone**, such as cortisol or glucagon, as part of its inbuilt fight or flight mechanism. This reaction helps us to act fast, defend ourselves in dangerous situations or make quick decisions. Our body releases **extra glucose into the blood** to enable our muscles to move fast and in turn our blood glucose levels rise. This reaction is natural but it is when we put ourselves under constant stress that the continual release of these hormones can begin doing damage, **raising our blood glucose levels** to the point where **insulin is non-effective**.

Stress is not only dangerous for people with diabetes but those with **pre-diabetes**. The release of stress hormones makes the pancreas work harder to release insulin and move the glucose from the blood to the muscle tissues. Eventually this can contribute to insulin resistance, which in turn can become diabetes. There are many people with stressful lives who do not develop diabetes but studies suggest **stress is a large contributor to diabetes** when coupled with **lifestyle** and **genetic factors**.

Finally, stress hormones such as **cortisol stimulate appetite**, that's right, stressing literally does make you eat more. Cortisol can also promote the **preservation of fat** around your abdomen, significantly increasing your risk of heart disease or heart attack. Any way you look at, stress is bad news for diabetics.

There are plenty of tactics you can adopt to keep your life as stress-free as possible.

- Sit down and reevaluate your schedule; how much of what you commit to each week is essential, and can you release yourself from any activities that steal precious time from you with little reward? You may need to be ruthless when it comes to social engagements that sap energy or people that agitate you; never feel bad for having to say no if it means avoiding a stressful situation.

- A long (or short if that's all you can commit to) soak in a hot bath with epsom salts will help melt the troubles of the world away. Alternatively, soak your feet in a foot spa or bucket with warm water and your favourite essential oil, such as lavender or ginger.

- Try popping an upbeat song on, cranking the volume up and just letting loose for three or four minutes to relieve tension.

- Take a gentle walk or hit the gym or pool to burn off any unwanted negative energy.

- Treat yourself to a movie date, either solo or with friends, and leave the stressful situation outside.

- Try your hand at meditation or mindful thinking. Search for one of the many free meditation apps available for both Apple and Android phones. Empty your mind, focus on your breathing and realign with what's truly important and truly beautiful in you and the world.

- **Yoga** is a great way to get active and reduce any stress you may be feeling. Yoga can not only lower your blood pressure but it can also help ease the symptoms of diabetes or help prevent complications from developing. As yoga and similar low-impact exercises **increase the circulation of blood** around the body it's perfect for diabetics who may be experiencing circulation problems and numbness in their arms or legs. There are basic poses you can try at home but never push yourself too hard without supervision, and if you experience any knee, back or joint problems it is best to **consult with a yoga instructor** before composing a routine.

5 Yoga Poses to Reduce Stress

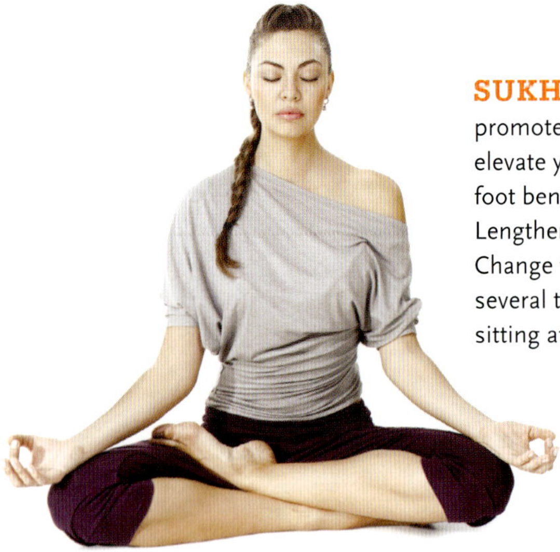

SUKHASANA (EASY POSE): A great meditative pose that promotes calm and also aligns the spine. Sit on a folded blanket to elevate your hips above your knees, cross your legs inwards (place each foot beneath the opposite knee) and place your hands on your knees. Lengthen your spine and relax your feet and thighs, hold for one minute. Change the cross of your legs and repeat. This is a great pose to perform several times a day, especially if you work in an office and are constantly sitting at a desk.

DOWNWARD FACING DOG: This is an easy pose for beginners and can help improve digestion and high blood pressure. For optimal benefit keep your fingers spread apart and your tummy tucked in. Start in a standing position with your arms by your side. As you exhale, keep your back straight and reach down to the floor, keeping your knees bent if needed and laying your palms flat on the ground. Step each foot back one at a time until you are in a push up pose, lift your hips up to create an inverted V then press your chest down toward your knees. Press your heels toward the floor and breathe deeply.

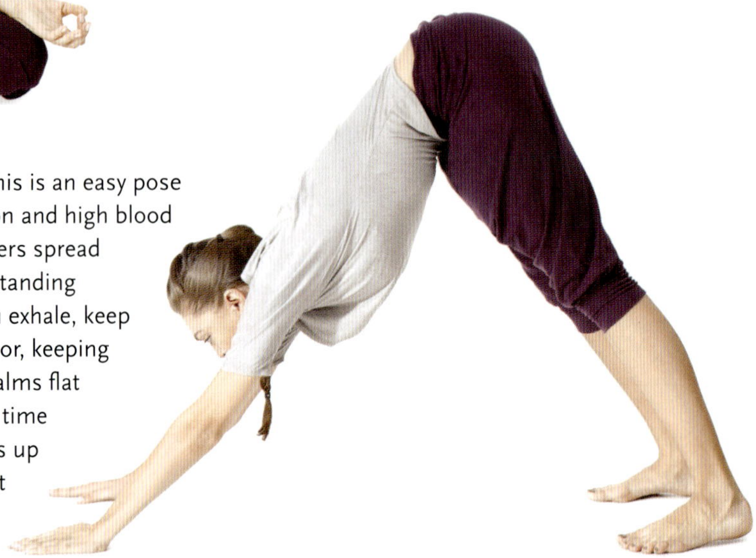

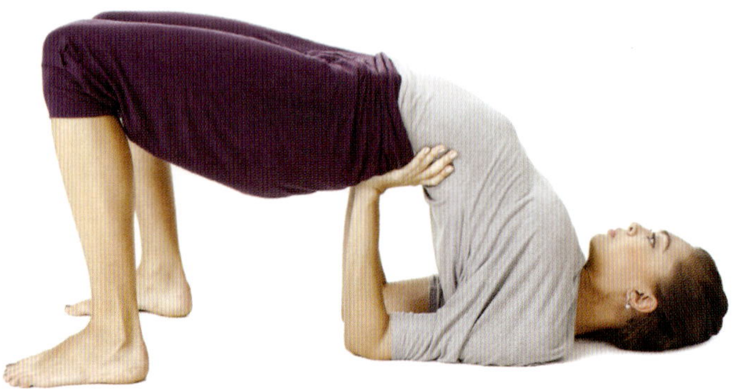

SETUBANDHASANA: This is a great pose for stretching the neck and spine; it also helps improve blood pressure and helps to relax the body and mind. Lie flat on the floor and as you exhale push with your feet and raise your body up. Make sure that your head and neck are flat on the floor. This pose shouldn't be overly-exertive and instead should be used for stretching and clearing the mind.

DHANURASANA (BOW POSE):

Begin by lying on your stomach with your arms by your side. Your feet should be hip-width apart. Fold your knees up towards your buttocks and hold your ankles. Breathe in and lift your chest off the ground as you pull your legs up and back so you feel yourself stretching like a bow and arrow. Focus on long, deep breaths and hold the pose for 20 – 30 seconds before releasing. This pose is great for strengthening your back, opening up the chest, and fighting stress and fatigue.

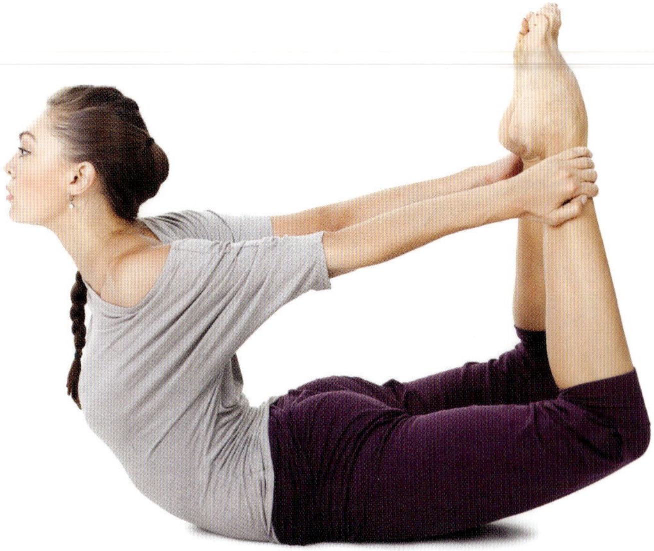

BHUJANGASANA (COBRA POSE):

To increase strength and flexibility in the arms, chest and back, the cobra pose is great to work into your daily routine and can be modified for beginners to the more advanced. When learning this pose, some people find it beneficial to place a pillow between their abdomen and chest to help support the movement and their back.

Lie on your stomach with your legs spread slightly apart and your hands flat on the floor next to your armpits, elbows should be pointed. Relax and inhale while pressing your hands into the floor and raising your chest and head off the ground. To protect your back, as you lift up, engage your abdominal muscles by drawing your belly button in towards your spine. Keep your legs and feet flat on the mat and stretch your upper body towards the ceiling, hold for 5 breaths before exhaling and lowering yourself slowly back onto the ground.

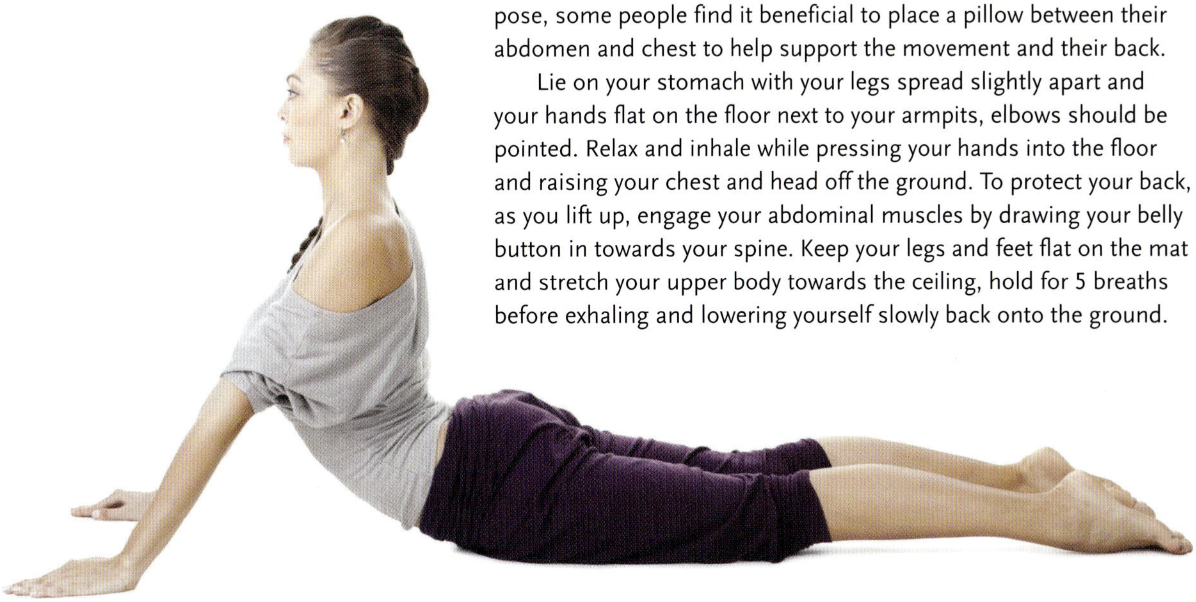

breakfast

Wok eggs with fresh greens
Sweet potato + bacon muffins
Sprouted lentil + artichoke bowl
Strawberry chia pudding
Pumpkin pie chia pudding
Brunch salad
Potato + leek hash browns
Super citrus granola with poached pear
Triple berry quinoa porridge

Wok eggs with fresh greens

Breakfast can be simple, speedy and nutritious with a little forward thinking. By cooking the eggs in the wok they are ready to eat in under a minute. Preparing the greens the night before and simply dressing before you eat is another way to ensure you make a healthier choice when pushed for time.

SERVES 2

4 free range eggs

2 spring onions/scallions, roughly chopped

Pinch of sea salt

A mix of watercress, baby spinach and rocket (arugula) leaves, rinsed and dried

1 avocado, sliced

¼ cup (60ml) extra virgin olive oil

¼ cup (60ml) fresh lemon juice

1 tbsp good quality seeded mustard

1 Heat a wok with 1 tbsp of coconut oil, swirl the oil around to coat halfway up the sides. Toss a few sea salt granules into the wok to see if it is hot enough, they should sizzle.

2 Crack the eggs into a bowl and give them a quick whisk before pouring into the wok. Working quickly, use a silicone spatula to move around the outside of the egg mixture, ensuring it doesn't stick to the wok. After 20 seconds, fold the egg mixture in half, as you would for an omelette. Loosen the bottom of the mixture and continue cooking for another 20–30 seconds before removing from the wok and setting aside.

3 Add the rinsed greens to a bowl with the sliced avocado. In a small bowl or jug whisk the extra virgin olive oil, lemon juice and mustard together before pouring over the greens. Serve the eggs alongside the greens and avocado.

Quick, simple and healthy breakfasts are the key to starting the day with a bang and set you up for better food choices and stable blood glucose levels.

Sweet potato + bacon muffins

Try these savoury sweet potato and bacon muffins that are delicious hot or cold, and give you a head start on hitting your daily vegetable quota. Serve with a smear of butter or try something different, such as ricotta or smashed avocado.

MAKES 6

½ cup (65g) brown rice flour

½ cup (50g) almond meal/flour

½ tsp baking powder

2 tsp ground cinnamon

3 free range eggs

½ cup (125ml) coconut oil, melted

¼ cup (60ml) rice malt syrup (optional)

1 medium sweet potato

1 small zucchini/courgette

1 tsp sea salt

½ tsp black pepper

2 bacon rashers, any cut

1 Preheat the oven to 180°C/350°F and place 6 liners in a muffin tin.

2 Sift flours, baking powder and cinnamon into a bowl, set aside.

3 Whisk eggs, coconut oil and rice malt syrup (if using) together and fold through the dry mixture.

4 Grate the sweet potato and zucchini, season with salt and pepper and add to the mixture. Add a little more coconut oil if the mixture is too dry.

5 Divide the batter between the muffin liners.

6 Dice the bacon and sprinkle evenly over the top of each muffin.

7 Bake in the oven for 40 minutes or until an inserted skewer comes out clean.

Sprouted lentil + artichoke bowl

This salad makes a refreshing change from the typical idea of what breakfast can be. If you're not keen on sprouting your own lentils right away, you can buy them from specialty produce stores and some supermarkets. Top the bowl with a cooked egg for a protein boost.

SERVES 1

SPROUTED LENTILS

2 cups (400g) dried lentils of choice

Glass jar

Muslin or breathable cloth to cover the jar

1 Prepare the sprouted lentils ahead of time by soaking them in filtered water overnight, or for up to 14 hours. Rinse the lentils thoroughly and drain any excess liquid. Place the lentils in a glass jar and cover the top with muslin cloth, secure with a rubber band. Store the jar on the kitchen counter and rinse the lentils once a day in water, making sure to drain any water before returning the lentils to the jar.

2 The lentils should begin sprouting after 3 days. Test one is ready before rinsing the lentils for a final time. Return the lentils to the jar, secure the cloth on top and store in the refrigerator for up to two weeks. If the lentils are slimy or smell off-putting, bin the batch and start again.

ARTICHOKE BOWL

1 cup (200g) sprouted lentils

½ cup (100g) artichoke hearts (store-bought in brine is fine)

1 inch piece of fresh ginger, grated

Juice and zest of ½ a lemon

Pinch of sea salt and black pepper

1 free range egg (optional)

1 In a small bowl combine the lentils, artichokes, fresh ginger, lemon juice and zest. Stir, taste and adjust seasoning with sea salt and black pepper.

2 Cook the egg to your liking (if using) and serve on top of the salad.

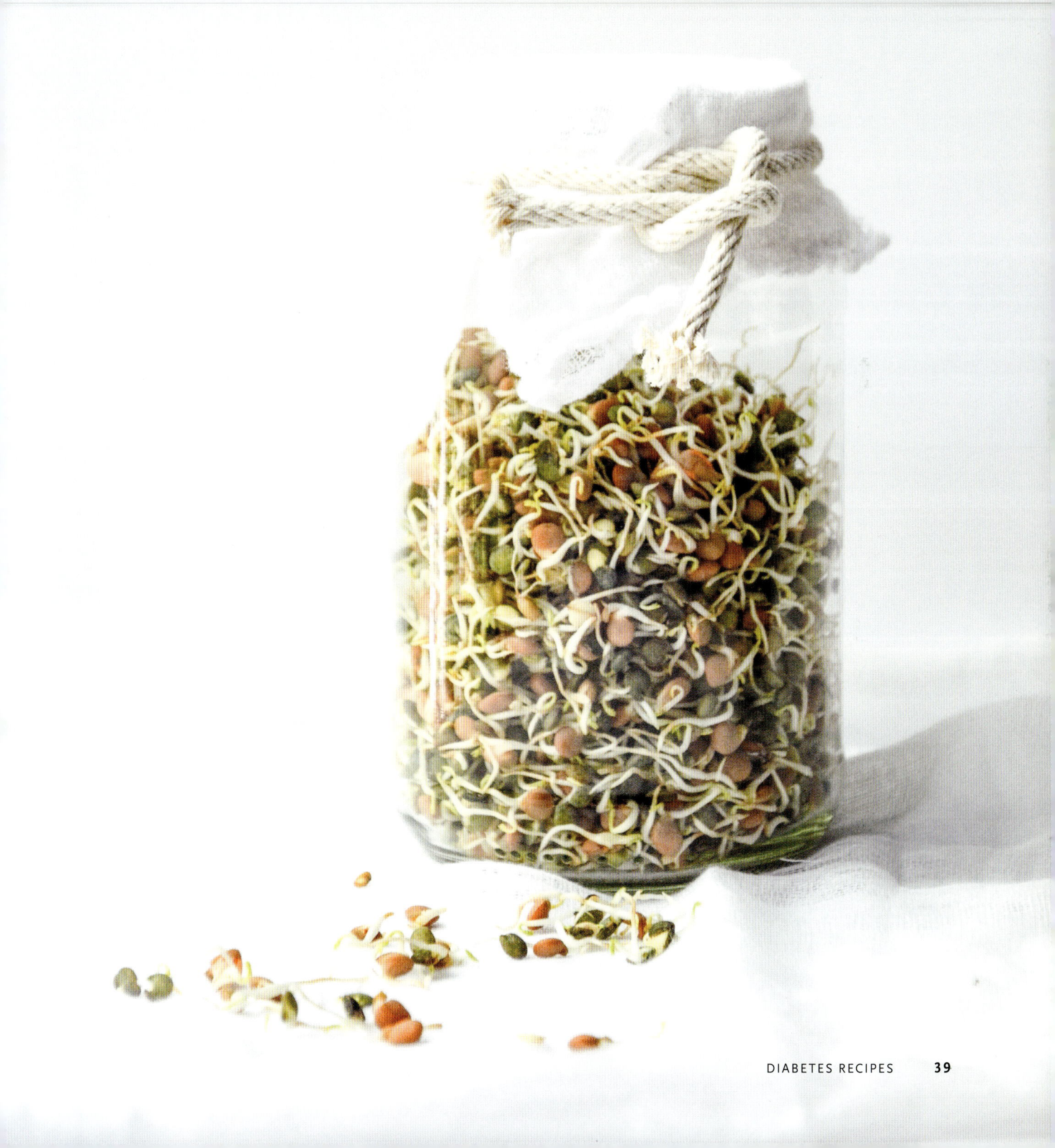

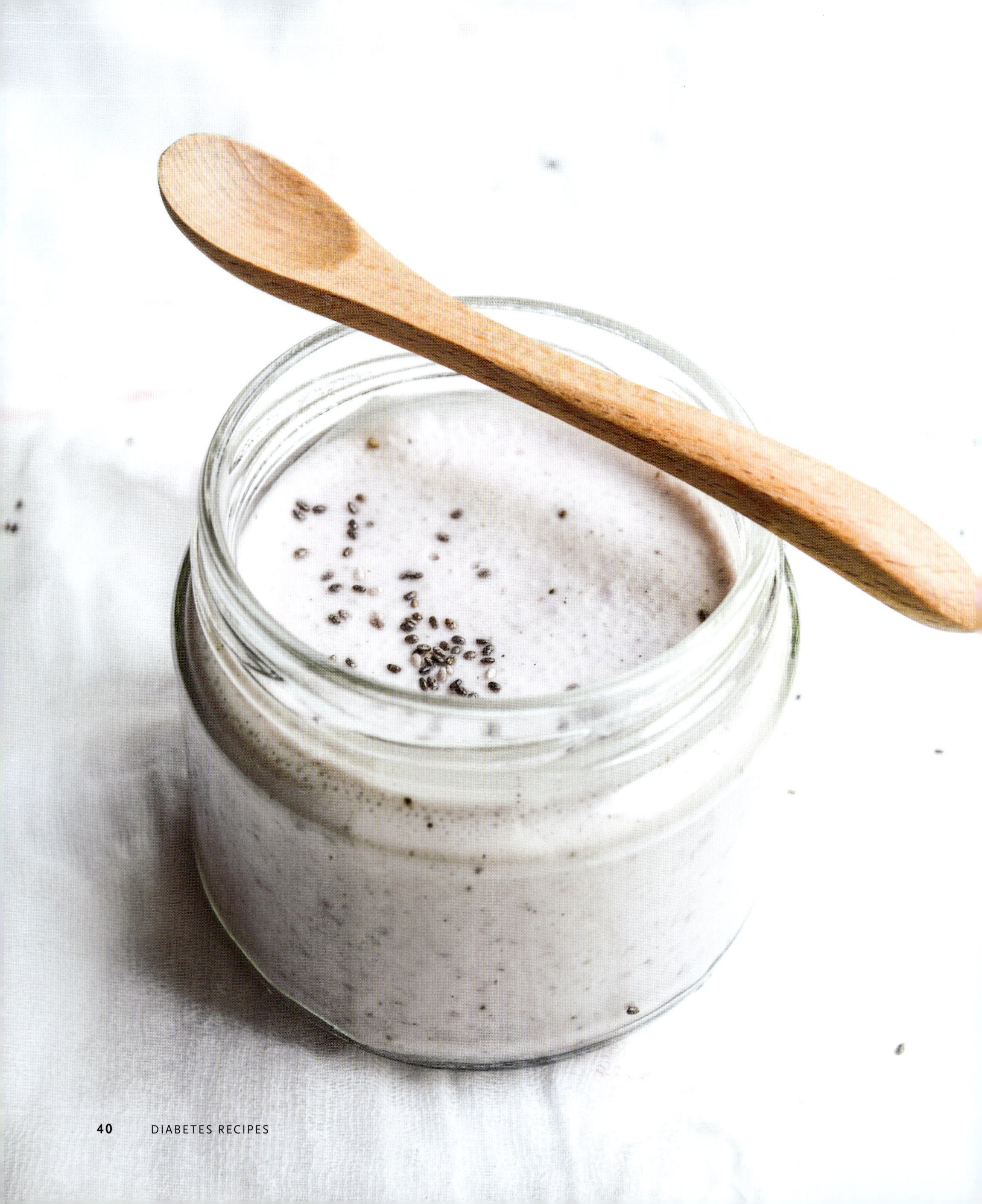

Strawberry chia pudding

This make-ahead breakfast is refreshing in the warmer months when seasonal fruit is at its ripest. Berries work great here or you could stew some stone fruit or apples in cinnamon then mix through the milk and chia seeds for a different flavour and texture.

SERVES 1

1 cup (250ml) coconut milk, full fat milk or any nut milk

1 cup (130g) fresh or frozen strawberries

½ cup (80g) shredded coconut

1 tbsp rice malt syrup or sweetener of choice (optional)

½ tsp vanilla powder

1 tsp cinnamon

2 tbsp chia seeds

In a blender or with a handheld immersion blender, puree milk, strawberries, shredded coconut, rice malt syrup (if using) and vanilla powder. Transfer the mixture to a bowl and whisk in the cinnamon and chia seeds. Place in the refrigerator for one hour to set. Serve at room temperature or chilled, topped with extra coconut and strawberries if desired.

Chia seeds are packed full of calcium, magnesium, fibre, omega 3s, manganese and phosphorus. The high level of antioxidants in chia seeds stops the crop from going rancid and a small amount in your diet each day or two goes a long way.

Pumpkin pie chia pudding

This is a sweet and creamy start to any day without the refined sugar hit that will see you slump before lunchtime. Make the pudding mixture ahead of time and divide between small jars. Store in the refrigerator and grab as a breakfast or snack on the run.

SERVES 4

1 cup (250ml) coconut milk, full fat milk or any nut milk

1 cup (225g) pumpkin or sweet potato puree

½ cup (40g) shredded coconut

1 tbsp rice malt syrup or sweetener of choice (optional)

½ tsp vanilla powder

1 tsp cinnamon

2 tbsp chia seeds

MAPLE ROASTED PECANS

⅓ cup (40g) pecans

1 tbsp maple syrup

¼ tsp ground cinnamon

1 In a blender or using a handheld immersion blender, puree the milk, pumpkin puree, shredded coconut, rice malt syrup and vanilla powder. Transfer the mixture to a bowl and whisk in the cinnamon and chia seeds. Place in the refrigerator for one hour to set.

2 To make the maple roasted pecans, preheat the oven to 160°C/320°F and line an oven tray with baking paper. Scatter the pecans over the tray and pour the maple syrup and cinnamon over the top, toss to coat. Roast in the oven for 5–10 minutes until browned. Set aside.

3 Serve at room temperature or chilled, topped with the maple roasted nuts and extra coconut if desired.

TIP: You can add more chia seeds to the pumpkin pie mix before setting for a thicker consistency depending on your preference.

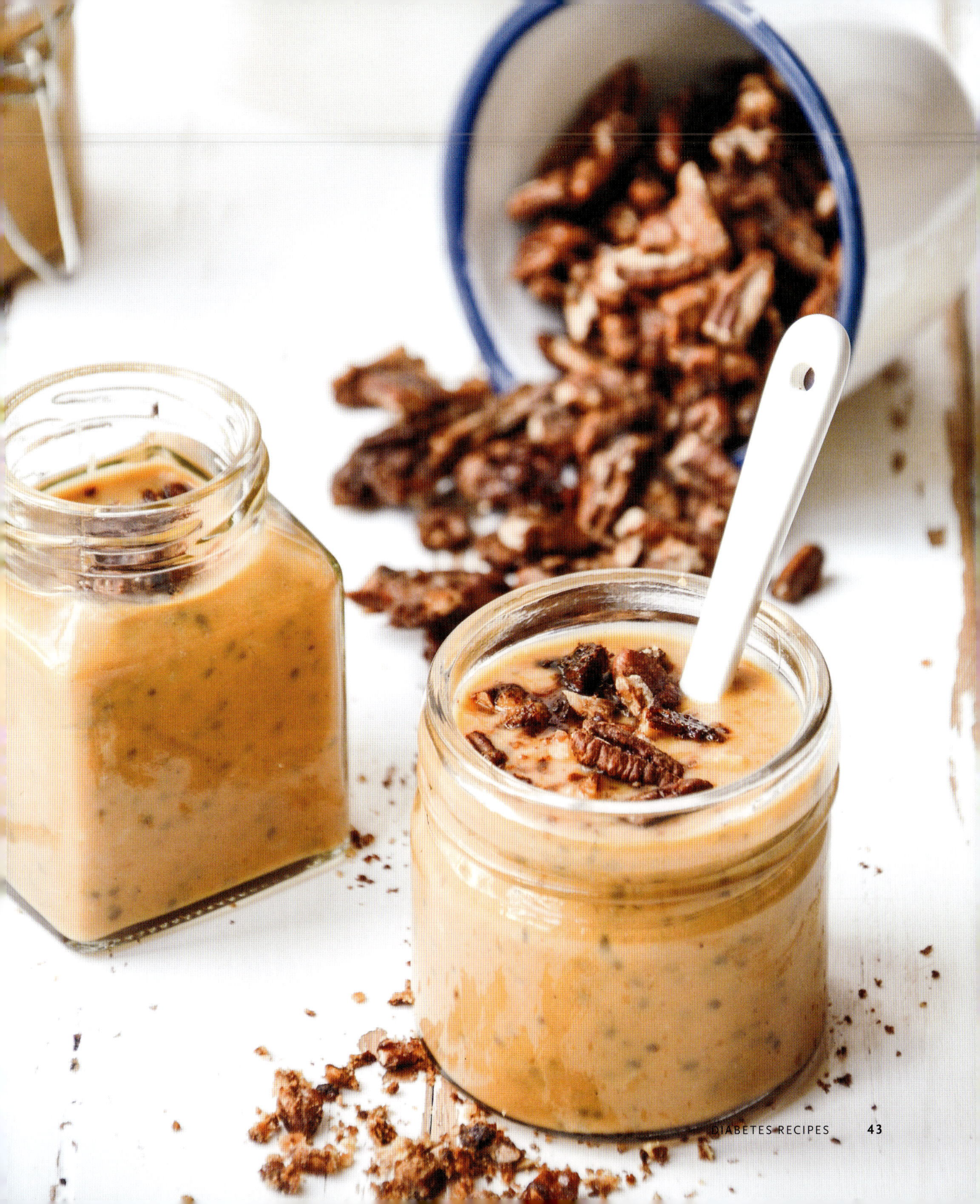

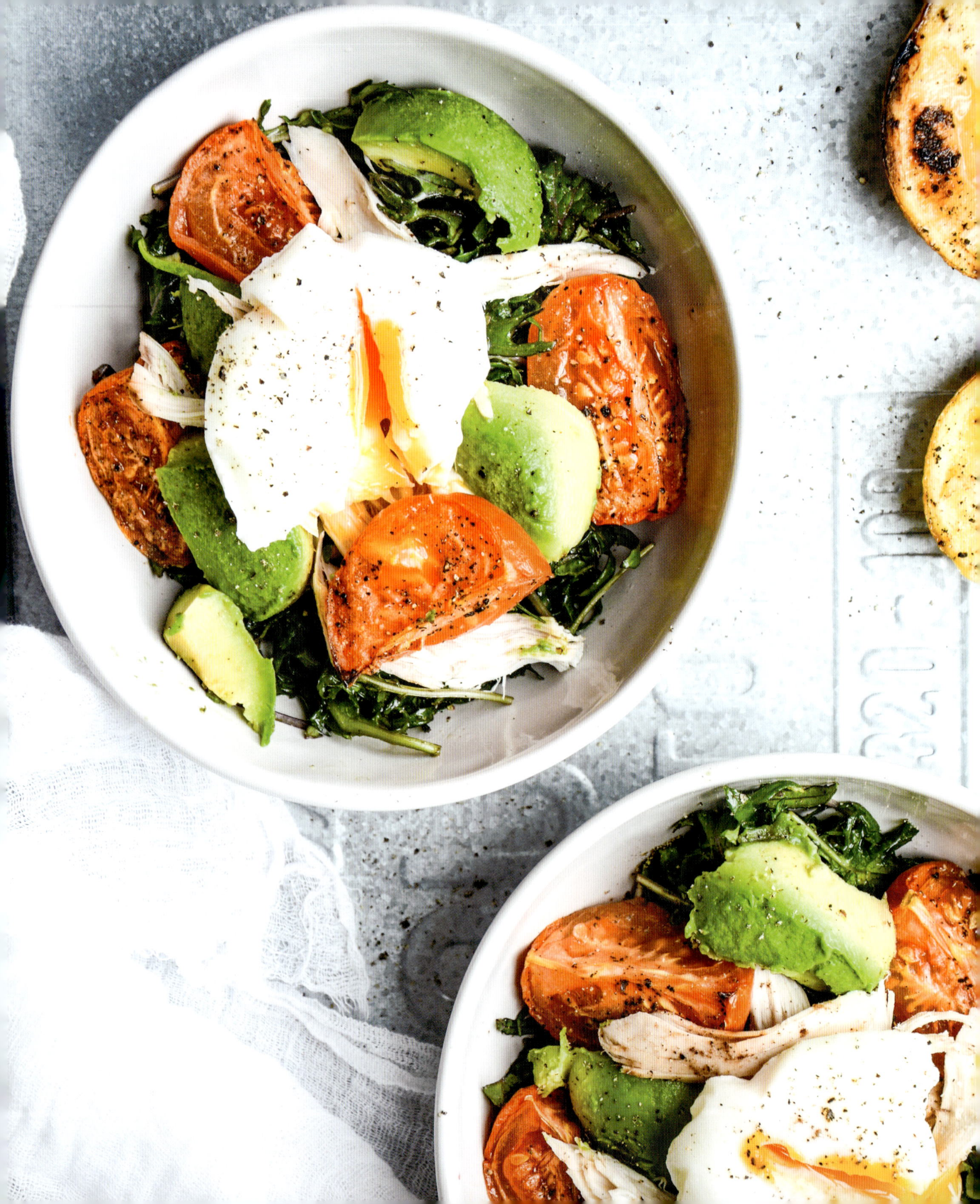

Brunch salad

Despite being called a brunch salad, this can be eaten at any time of the day. You can substitute any leafy green for the kale (such as spinach) and interchange your protein (exchange chicken for canned tuna or leftover roast meat from last night's dinner); there are no rules, use what you love or simply what's in your refrigerator.

SERVES 2 – 4

3 tomatoes

1 lemon

1 medium bunch (approximately 450g/1lb) of kale, stems removed

4 free range eggs

250g/9 oz chicken breast fillet, thinly sliced

1 avocado

LEMON DILL SAUCE

2 tbsp extra virgin olive oil

2 tbsp fresh lemon juice

1 tbsp finely chopped dill

Sea salt and black pepper to taste

1 Pre-heat the oven to 180°C/350°F. Thickly slice the tomatoes and lemon into rounds or wedges and lay on a lined baking tray. Drizzle with olive or coconut oil, season with salt and pepper and roast in the oven for 20 minutes or until cooked to your liking. Remove and let cool.

2 Prepare the lemon dill sauce by whisking all ingredients together in a bowl or jug.

3 Discard the kale stems and cut the leaves into chunks, transfer to a small bowl. Pour over half the lemon dill sauce and use your hands to massage it into the leaves until tender, approximately 2 minutes. If you are using baby kale, simply pour the sauce over the leaves and toss gently.

4 Place eggs in a small saucepan and cover with cold water. Bring to the boil and cook the eggs to your liking (2 minutes for a soft boiled egg, 4–5 minutes for medium boiled, depending on the size of the eggs). Once the eggs have cooled, peel the shell off. Alternatively, poach the eggs in a saucepan of simmering water for runny yolks.

5 Slice the chicken breast into thin strips and heat up a small frying pan. Season the chicken with a pinch of black pepper. Add a drizzle of extra virgin olive oil and cook the chicken for 5 minutes, cutting into a strip to check it is cooked through before removing all of the chicken and setting it aside. Alternatively, use roast chicken (store bought or home cooked) and shred the chicken breast meat into strips.

6 Slice the avocado to desired thickness.

7 Assemble the salad starting with the kale, adding the avocado, eggs, roasted tomato, chicken, and finishing with the remaining lemon dill sauce and juice from the roasted lemon.

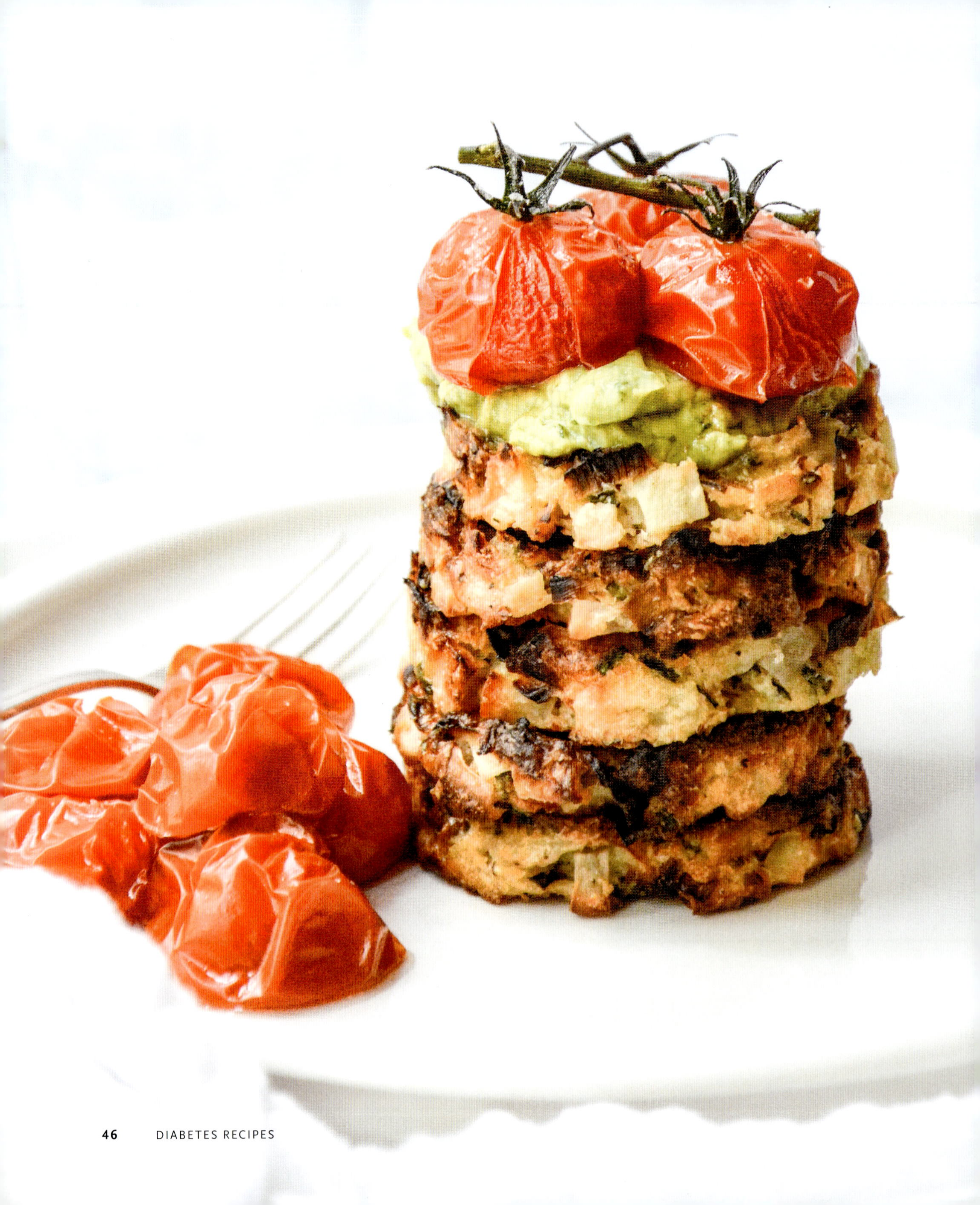

Potato + leek hash browns

These baked hash browns are a real crowd pleaser, don't require too much prep work and can be topped with an endless array of ingredients. Make a batch ahead of time and freeze in individual portions then simply reheat in the oven.

MAKES 8

4 medium potatoes

1 leek

25g/1 oz butter

½ cup (65g) rice flour

Sea salt and black pepper

CORIANDER GUACAMOLE

1 large avocado

Juice of ½ a lemon

Handful of coriander/cilantro leaves

Pinch of sea salt

1 Preheat the oven to 180°C/350°F and line an oven tray with baking paper. Peel the potatoes and cut each into even cubes. Steam the potatoes for 4–5 minutes, either in a microwave or in a steamer basket on the stovetop over simmering water. The potato should be tender but still hold its shape. Take half the mixture and puree it then stir through the rest of the potato so you have a mixture of smooth and chunky potato.

2 Clean the leek and dice into even chunks. In a small pan, cook the leek in butter until soft. Set aside to cool slightly then stir through the potato mixture with the rice flour and a good pinch of sea salt and black pepper for flavour.

3 Using an egg ring placed on the oven tray as a guide, spoon the mixture into the egg ring and push down until flat. Remove the egg ring carefully, reposition it further along the tray and repeat the process until you have used up all of the mixture. Bake in the oven for 30 minutes or until golden brown.

4 Prepare the guacamole by blitzing the avocado, lemon juice, coriander and sea salt in a food processor until smooth. Serve the guacamole on top of the hash browns along with any additional toppings such as roasted cherry tomatoes.

Super citrus granola with poached pear

A tasty alternative to store-bought cereal or granola, you can also control the flavour and amount of sweetener added when you make your own. This zingy combination of lemon and grapefruit zest and juice is complimented by the spiciness of nutmeg and ginger, making it a warming start to the day. Serve with a poached pear or fruit of choice.

SERVES 1

1 cup (100g) rolled oats
¼ cup (20g) shredded coconut
2 tbsp coconut oil, melted
1 tbsp rice malt syrup (optional)
Zest of 1 lemon
Zest of 1 grapefruit
1 tbsp lemon juice
1 tbsp grapefruit juice
1 tsp ground nutmeg
1 tsp ground ginger

1 pear
½ tsp vanilla powder
½ tsp cinnamon

1 Preheat the oven to 180°C/350°F and line a baking tray with baking paper.

2 Combine rolled oats, shredded coconut, coconut oil, rice malt syrup (if using), lemon and grapefruit zest and juice, nutmeg and ginger in a bowl.

3 Spread the mixture evenly over the lined tray and bake in the oven for 10–15 minutes or until golden brown, careful not to let it burn.

4 Remove from the oven, let cool and store in an airtight container.

5 Bring a small saucepan of water with a squeeze of lemon juice in it to the boil then reduce to a simmer. Peel the pear's skin off from the stem down and lower into the water. Add the vanilla powder and poach the pear for 15–20 minutes until soft.

6 Serve granola with milk or natural yoghurt, topped with poached pear and a sprinkling of lemon zest.

Grapefruit can interact negatively with some diabetes medications. Check with your doctor beforehand or simply replace with lime zest and juice.

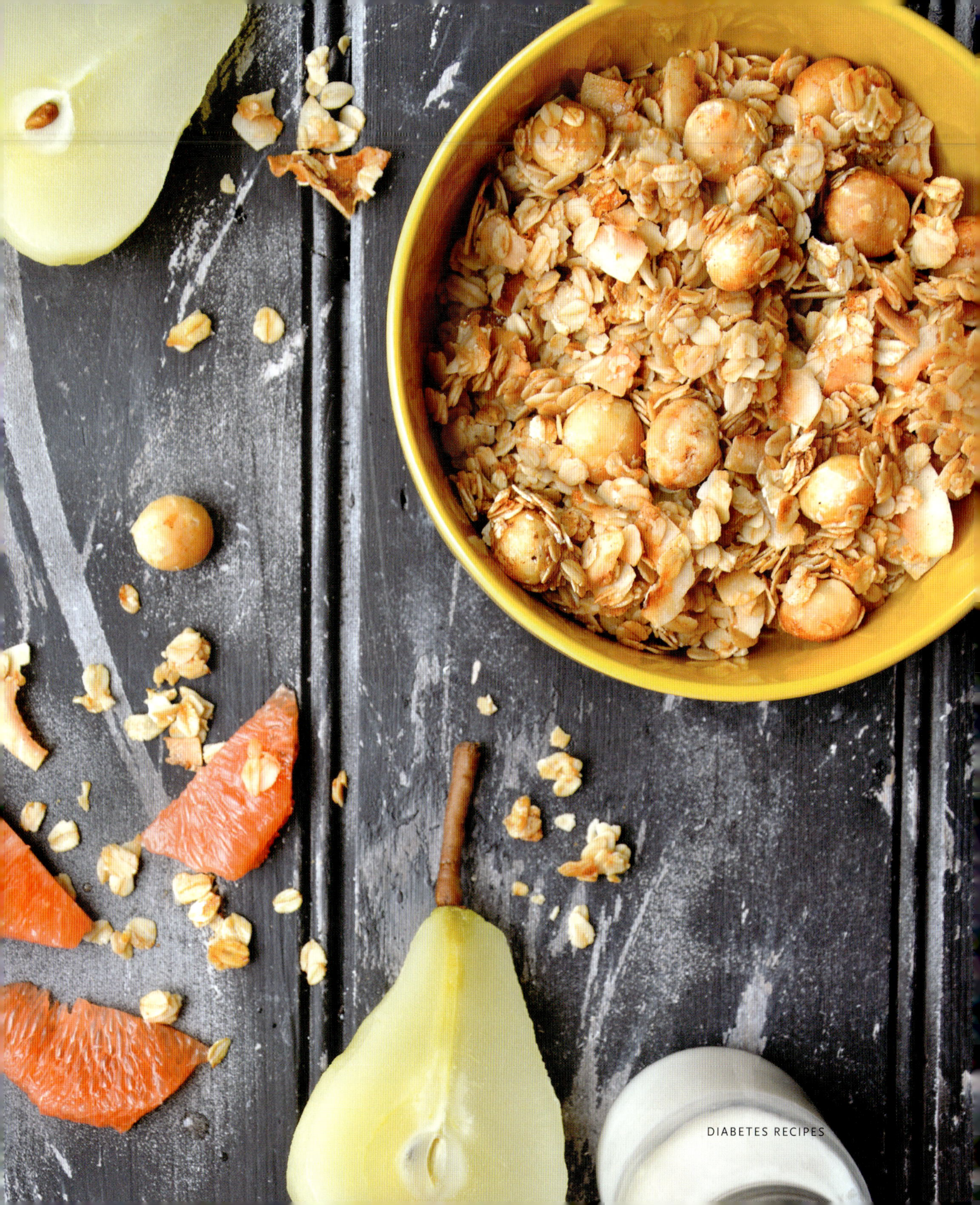

Triple berry quinoa porridge

This is a great recipe to use up leftover quinoa and is a different yet easy spin on the traditional oat porridge. The burst of flavours the berries and coconut offer is a welcome start to any day and the inclusion of cinnamon is a great blood sugar stabiliser to include in your daily diet.

SERVES 1

- **⅔ cup (80g) cooked quinoa**
- **¼ cup (60g) natural yoghurt (or coconut milk)**
- **1 tbsp unsweetened shredded coconut**
- **Pinch of cinnamon**
- **Handful of blueberries, raspberries and blackberries**
- **8 almonds (pre-soaked overnight and chopped)**

1. In a bowl combine the quinoa with yoghurt, shredded coconut and cinnamon to taste.
2. Top porridge with berries and chopped almonds.
3. If extra sweetness is desired add a sweetener of choice, either a small amount of local raw honey, rice malt syrup or one date.

Soak the almonds overnight in a bowl of filtered water to "activate" them. This process helps removes the enzyme inhibitor in the nut's skin and allows your body to digest it better while also reaping more of the nut's nutrients. When ready to serve, rinse the nuts thoroughly in filtered water.

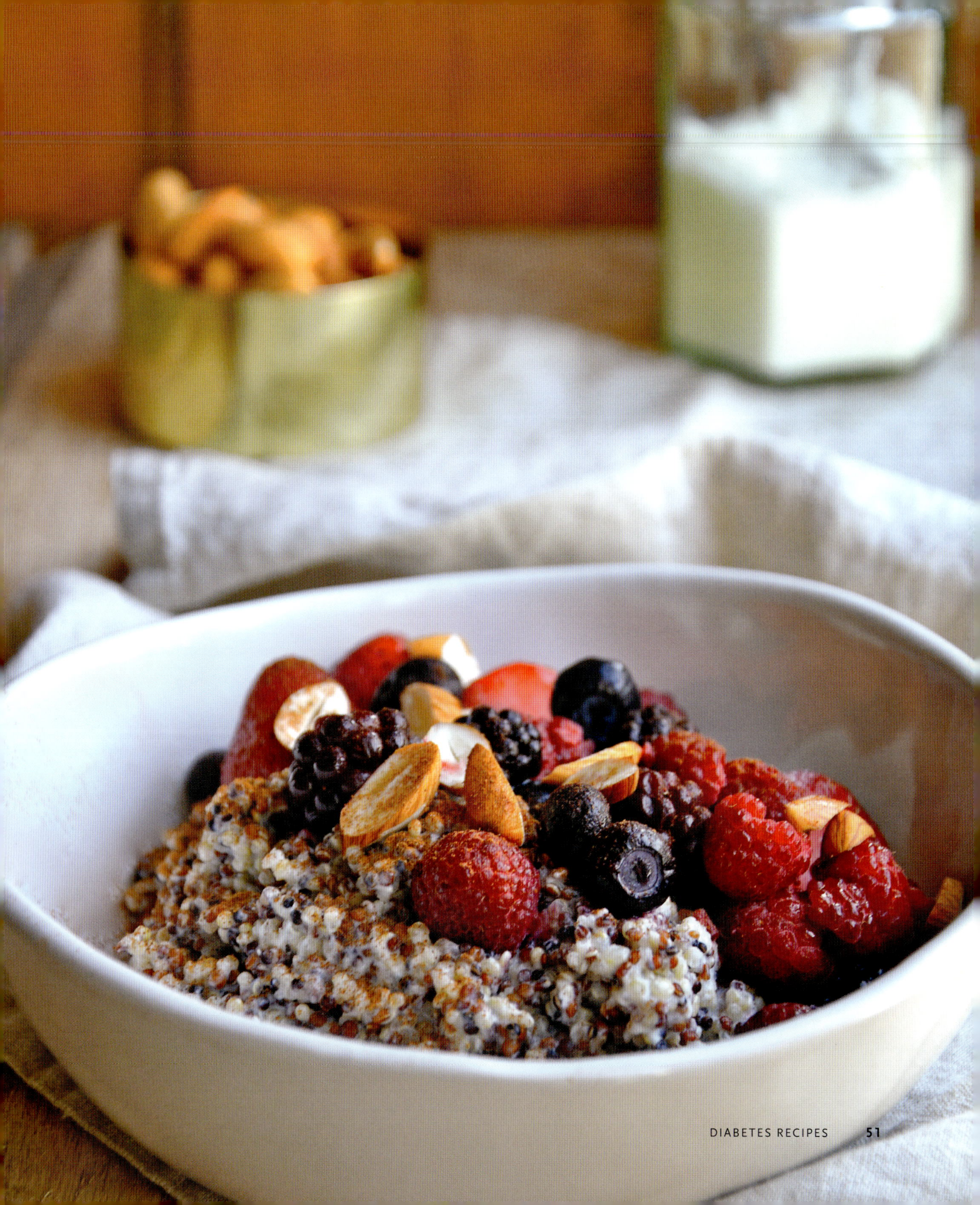

salads & sides

Carrot + black sesame salad
Choose your greens salad
Garlic stir fried broccoli + green beans
Fresh freekeh salad
Roasted Brussels sprouts with tahini dressing
Simple tuna salad
Avocado, haloumi + raspberry salad
Simple coleslaw
Cauliflower tabouli
Chilli pumpkin + goat cheese spread
Zucchini hummus
Lemon hummus
Avocado white bean smash
Baba ganoush dip
Basic sauerkraut
Simple kim chi
Peach, prosciutto + goat cheese rolls
Pepita crusted chicken strips
Potato wedges with guacamole
Prawn + sprouts rice paper rolls

Carrot + black sesame salad

I feel like carrots often don't make the cut when it comes to salads. This recipe will transform the way you think of a carrot salad. It's incredibly easy and quick to prepare, with minimal dressing and fuss.

SERVES 6

2 large orange carrots

2 large yellow carrots

100g/3.5 oz good quality goat cheese (marinated in extra virgin olive oil if possible)

¼ cup (35g) black sesame seeds

1 Peel the carrots and trim the ends. Using a julienne peeler, slice the carrots into thin strands. A julienne peeler is a cheap addition to your kitchen but is not a necessity. You can finely slice the carrot with a knife but this will of course take longer and may yield different results.

2 Add the carrots to a serving bowl or platter, piled high. Dot the salad with chunks of goat cheese and drizzle some of the marinating oil over the salad. If the goat cheese you are using didn't come in oil, simply drizzle some extra virgin olive oil over the top.

3 Sprinkle the black sesame seeds over the top of the salad and serve. If you can't locate black sesame seeds you can replace with regular sesame seeds, which should be available at all supermarkets.

Choose your greens salad

SERVES 6

450g/1 lb mixed greens of choice

1 large avocado

1 large cucumber

Thoroughly rinse and dry the greens and add to a large bowl. Slice the avocado and cucumber and add to the greens.

CHOOSE YOUR DRESSING

KEEP IT SIMPLE

Scatter freshly chopped dill and a handful of pepitas (pumpkin seeds) over the top then toss through. Drizzle olive oil over before serving.

SUPER GREENS

Puree ½ an avocado with the juice of 1 lemon, a good pinch of sea salt, and enough water to thin the dressing out to a pourable consistency. Drizzle over and toss through before serving.

BIT OF A BITE

Whisk together ¼ cup (60ml) of apple cider vinegar with 1 tbsp of rice wine vinegar and 2 crushed garlic cloves. Whisk in extra virgin olive oil to desired consistency and toss through the salad before serving.

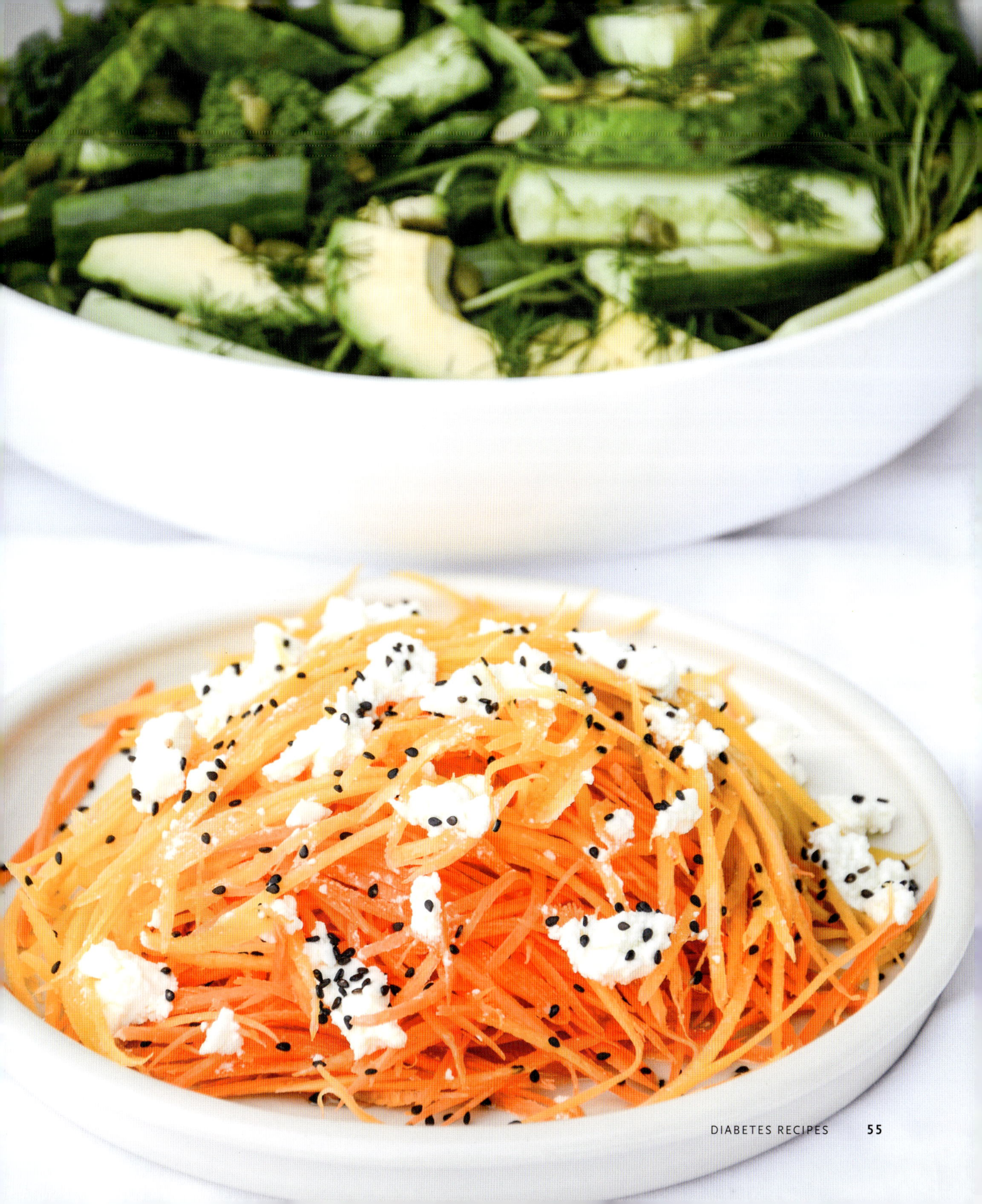

Garlic stir fried broccoli + green beans

Stir frying vegetables until just cooked but still crisp is a great way to add texture to a meal. This cooking method also allows you to experiment with Asian flavours that you may not usually consider. Try adding sesame oil, chilli flakes or lemongrass to the garlic for a flavour boost, or substituting the broccoli for some Asian greens.

SERVES 2

2 cups (180g) broccoli florets
1 cup (60–80g) green (string) beans
4 garlic cloves
Extra virgin olive oil
1 tsp ground turmeric
1 tsp ground cumin
Pinch of sea salt and black pepper

1 Cut the broccoli into florets and top and tail the green beans, cutting them in half if they are large.

2 Peel the garlic cloves and use the flat side of a knife to push down on the clove and smash it open.

3 Heat 1 tbsp of coconut oil in a pan or wok over high heat and add the broccoli, beans and garlic cloves.

4 Stir fry the vegetables for 3–4 minutes before adding the ground turmeric, cumin, sea salt and black pepper. Remove from the heat while the broccoli and beans still have a slight crunch to them.

Bulk this side dish up by adding strips of chicken or beef to create a full meal. Add another vegetable, such as a couple of bulbs of bok choy, a good drizzle of sesame oil or tamari (soy sauce) to help flavour the chicken, and sprinkle sesame seeds over the top before serving. Simple, fast and fresh.

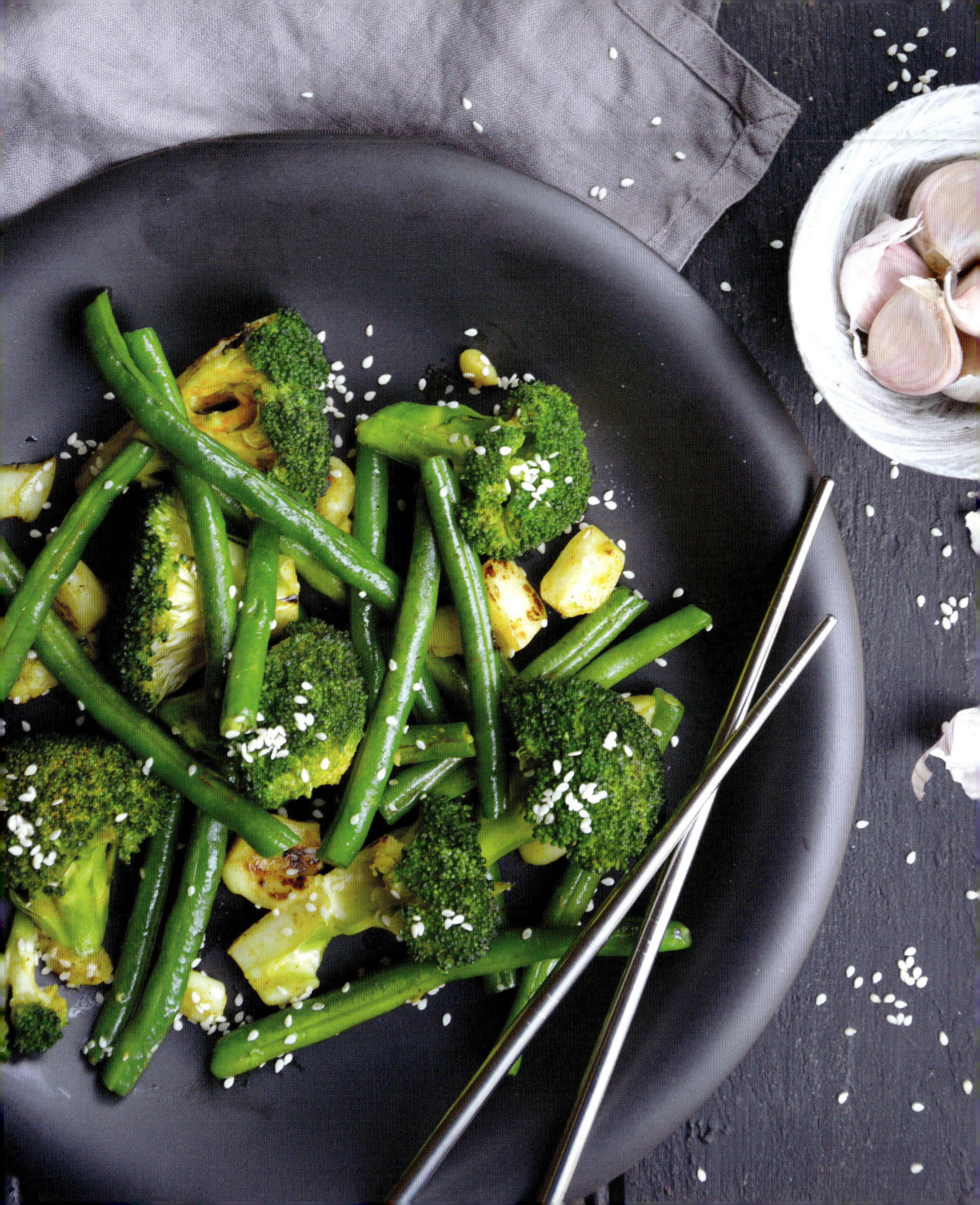

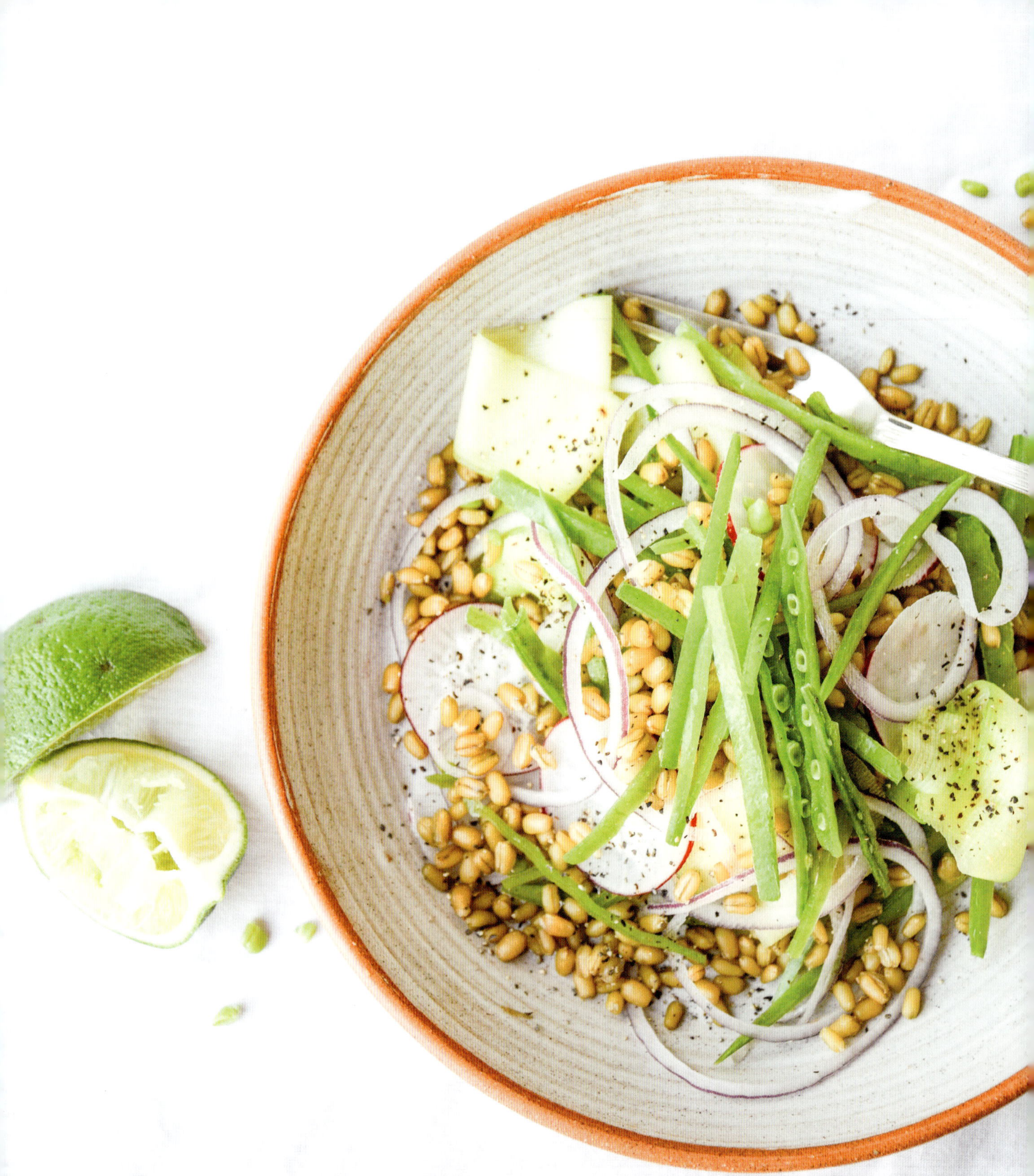

Fresh freekeh salad

Freekeh is young, green wheat and can be a great source of fibre in your diet. As with all ingredients, it's best to try it and see how your body and blood sugar respond before adding it to your regular menu. Freekeh is also a great source of protein, potassium and magnesium, and can be enjoyed warm or served cold in salads. There are two varieties of freekeh you can buy, cracked or uncracked. Cooking times will vary depending on which variety you buy: for uncracked freekeh simmer for 45–60 minutes until tender, for cracked freekeh the cooking time reduces to only 15–20 minutes.

SERVES 2

1 cup (180g) freekeh

2½ cups (750ml) water or stock of choice

2 tbsp extra virgin olive oil

Juice of 1 lime

Pinch of sea salt and black pepper

1 medium cucumber

½ Spanish/red onion

4 large red radishes

8 snow peas

1 Soak the freekeh in a bowl of filtered water overnight.

2 When ready to cook, drain the freekeh in fresh water and add to a saucepan with the water or stock. Simmer over medium heat until tender (see cooking times above), stir during cooking if needed. Drain the freekeh in a sieve to remove any remaining liquid then transfer to a bowl.

3 Whisk the olive oil, lemon juice and sea salt and pepper together. Set aside.

4 Cut the cucumber into ribbons using a vegetable peeler, or slice thinly with a knife.

5 Peel the onion and finely slice, along with the radishes and snow peas. Add the cucumber, onion, radishes and snow peas to the bowl of freekeh and pour the dressing over the top. Toss gently to mix the ingredients and serve.

Roasted Brussels sprouts with tahini dressing

Even the fussiest eater will be surprised by the flavour that roasting brings out in these Brussels sprouts, and the tahini dressing is so versatile, it's great drizzled over any vegetable.

SERVES 2

250g/9 oz Brussels sprouts

Extra virgin olive oil

2 tsp chilli flakes (optional)

Salt and pepper to taste

TAHINI DRESSING

2 tbsp hulled tahini

2 tbsp water (more as needed)

Zest and juice of ½ a lemon

1 tsp paprika

1 garlic clove, crushed (optional)

1 Preheat the oven to 180°C/350°F and line an oven tray with baking paper.

2 Trim the ends from the Brussels sprouts before coating in olive oil, chilli flakes, salt and pepper. Roast for approximately 20 minutes until brown, careful not to let them burn.

3 Prepare the dressing by whisking together the tahini, water, lemon zest, paprika and crushed garlic in a small bowl.

4 Serve the Brussels sprouts warm with the dressing over the top and optional chilli flakes for an added flavour hit.

If Brussels sprouts aren't your thing, try this recipe with a wedge of green cabbage. Not only is cabbage an extremely affordable option when you're trying to eat well on a budget but a little goes a long way. You'll be surprised at how the flavour and texture profile can change when you roast cabbage until slightly caramelised.

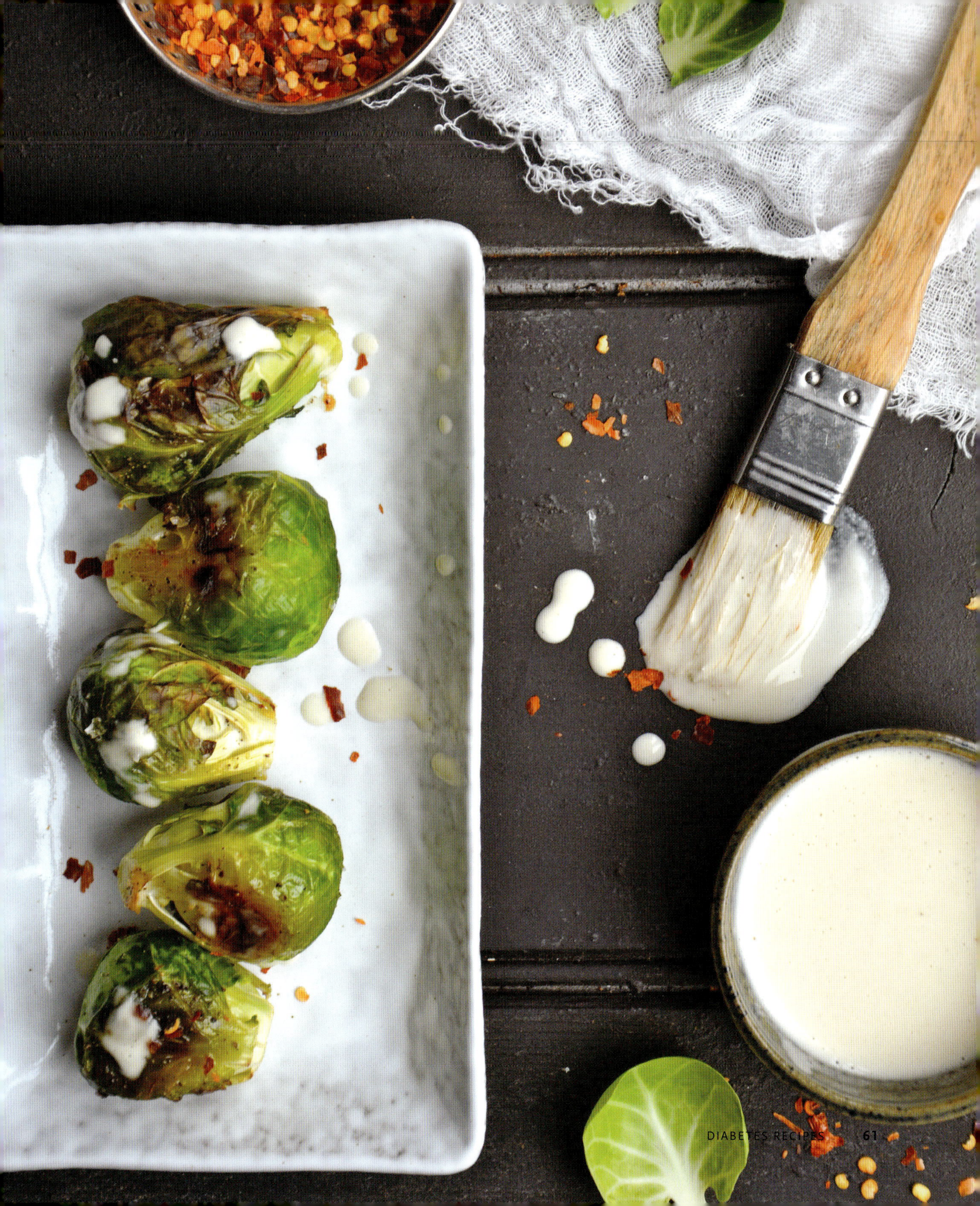

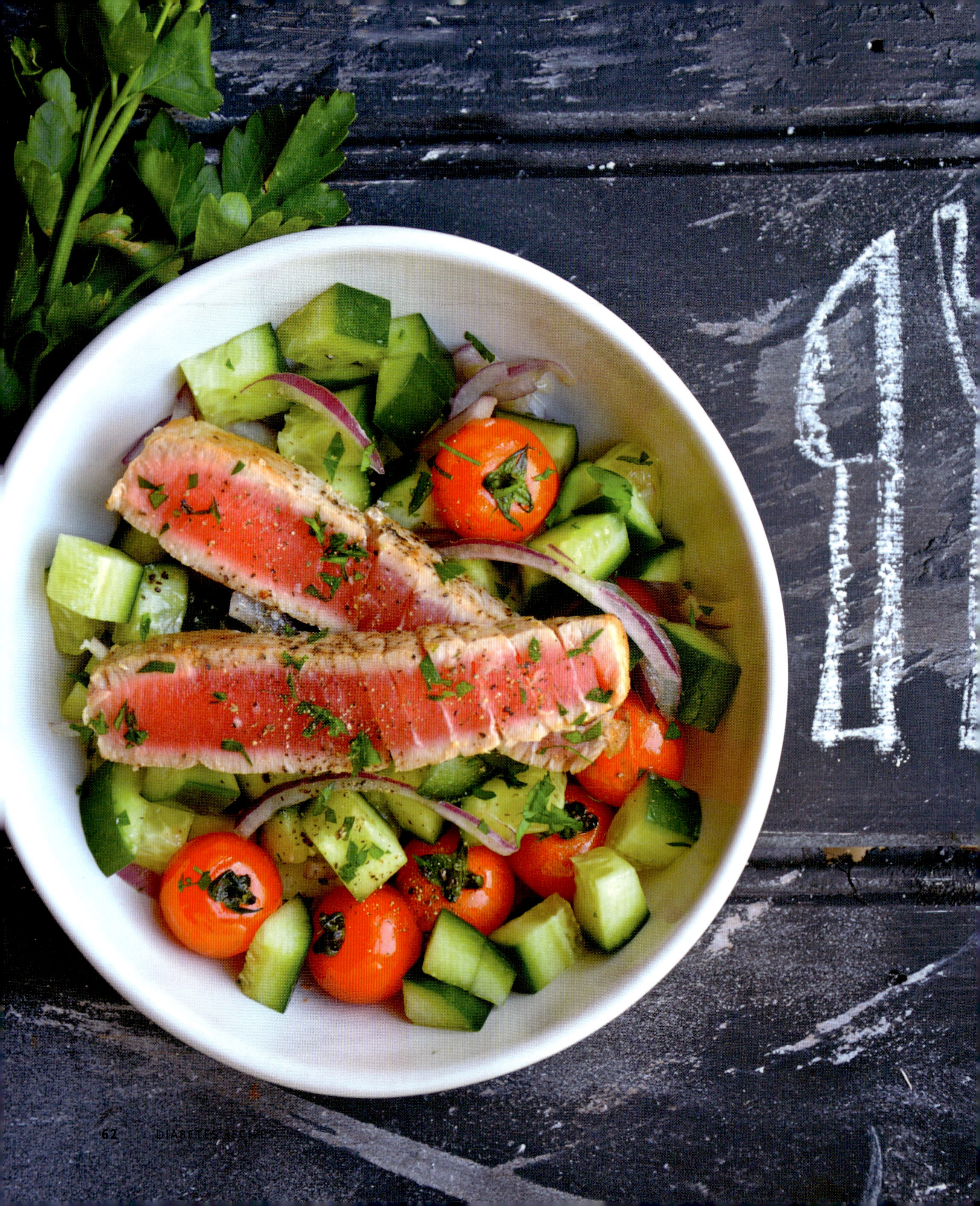

Simple tuna salad

When we think of a tuna salad, most of us envisage a can of tuna that we empty onto a plate with a few leaves and seasonings. It's not hard to cook a tuna steak at home if you have access to good quality fresh tuna, and it makes the world of difference in texture and taste. Keep the salad simple with seasoning so you can really appreciate the natural flavour of the fish.

SERVES 1

8 cherry tomatoes

1 small cucumber

¼ Spanish/red onion

Small fresh tuna steak (up to 150g/ 5 oz)

Sea salt and black pepper

Extra virgin olive oil

1 In a pan, drizzle a small amount of extra virgin olive oil and cook the cherry tomatoes for 3–4 minutes until the skin begins to darken and the tomatoes soften. Remove from the heat and set aside.

2 Dice the cucumber and finely slice the red onion.

3 Season both sides of the tuna steak with sea salt and black pepper; use your hands to gently press the seasoning into the flesh.

4 Heat a small pan with a drizzle of extra virgin olive oil. Lay the tuna steak into the hot pan and cook for 1–2 minutes each side. Set aside to rest for 4 minutes.

5 Slice the tuna steak and assemble the salad by laying the tuna on top of the tomatoes, cucumber and red onion. Drizzle a small amount of extra virgin olive oil over the top if desired.

The tuna in this recipe can be replaced with another fish, such as salmon, or a small chicken breast or beef fillet. Choose good quality produce to let the natural flavours shine and to minimise the need for excessive seasoning or sauces.

Avocado, haloumi + raspberry salad

This is such a great combination of flavours; it can be served alongside a protein of choice, such as chicken, or enjoyed on its own. The nutty avocado mixed with the sweet raspberries and salty haloumi ensures every mouthful of this salad is a delight.

SERVES 2

250g/9 oz haloumi, diced

1 ripe avocado, diced

250g/9 oz fresh raspberries

Extra virgin olive oil

1 tbsp fresh lemon juice

Sea salt and black pepper

1 In a small pan, cook the haloumi until brown. You may add a small drizzle of olive oil to help crisp the cheese up but it is not necessary.

2 Make the salad by combining diced avocado and fresh raspberries with the cooked haloumi. To bulk up the salad add bitter greens such as rocket (arugula).

3 Drizzle a small amount of extra virgin olive oil and fresh lemon juice over the top and season with a pinch of sea salt and a good grinding of fresh black pepper. Gently toss before serving.

Simple coleslaw

Here's a cheap and simple replacement for store bought coleslaw dressing that doesn't sacrifice on taste. Dress up your coleslaw with additional vegetables or keep it simple for a fuss-free salad.

SERVES 2-4

¼ red cabbage

¼ green cabbage

1 large carrot

Optional extras: spring onion/ scallion, any colour capsicum/ pepper, celery

DRESSING

3 tbsp hulled tahini

1 tbsp freshly minced garlic

Juice and zest of ½ a lemon

Pinch of sea salt and black pepper

1 Finely slice the red and green cabbage and set aside in a large bowl.

2 Wash the carrot or peel the skin off. Use a julienne slicer, a mandolin slicer or a knife to thinly slice the carrot into strips. Add to the bowl of cabbage.

3 In a small bowl or jar, combine the tahini, garlic, lemon juice and zest, and sea salt and black pepper. If using a jar, place the lid on and shake until emulsified. If using a bowl, whisk the mixture together. Taste and adjust seasoning if required.

4 Pour the dressing over the cabbage and carrot and use a pair of tongs to mix together until the dressing is evenly distributed. Serve immediately or refrigerate for 1–2 hours to allow the dressing to soften the cabbage and carrot slightly.

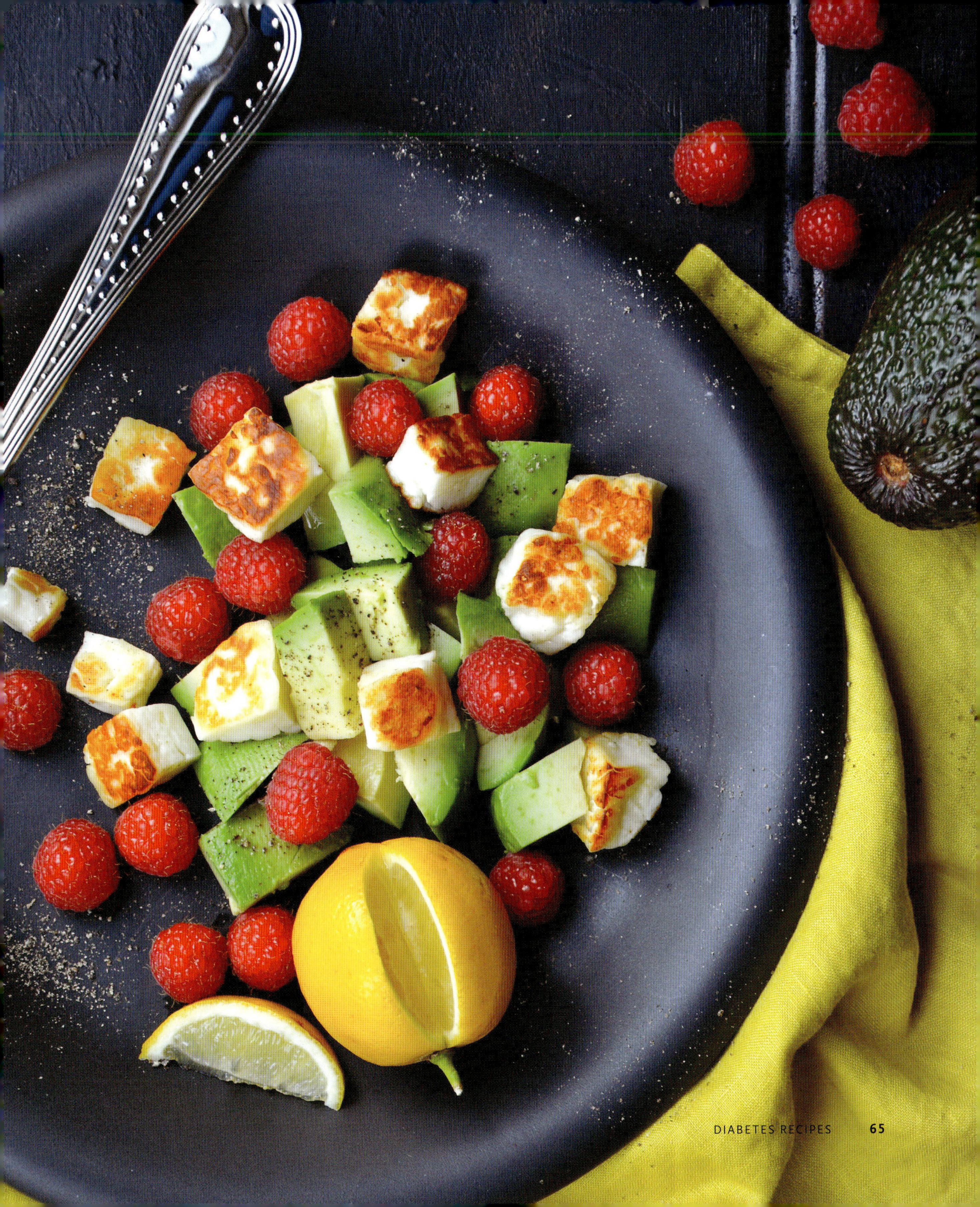

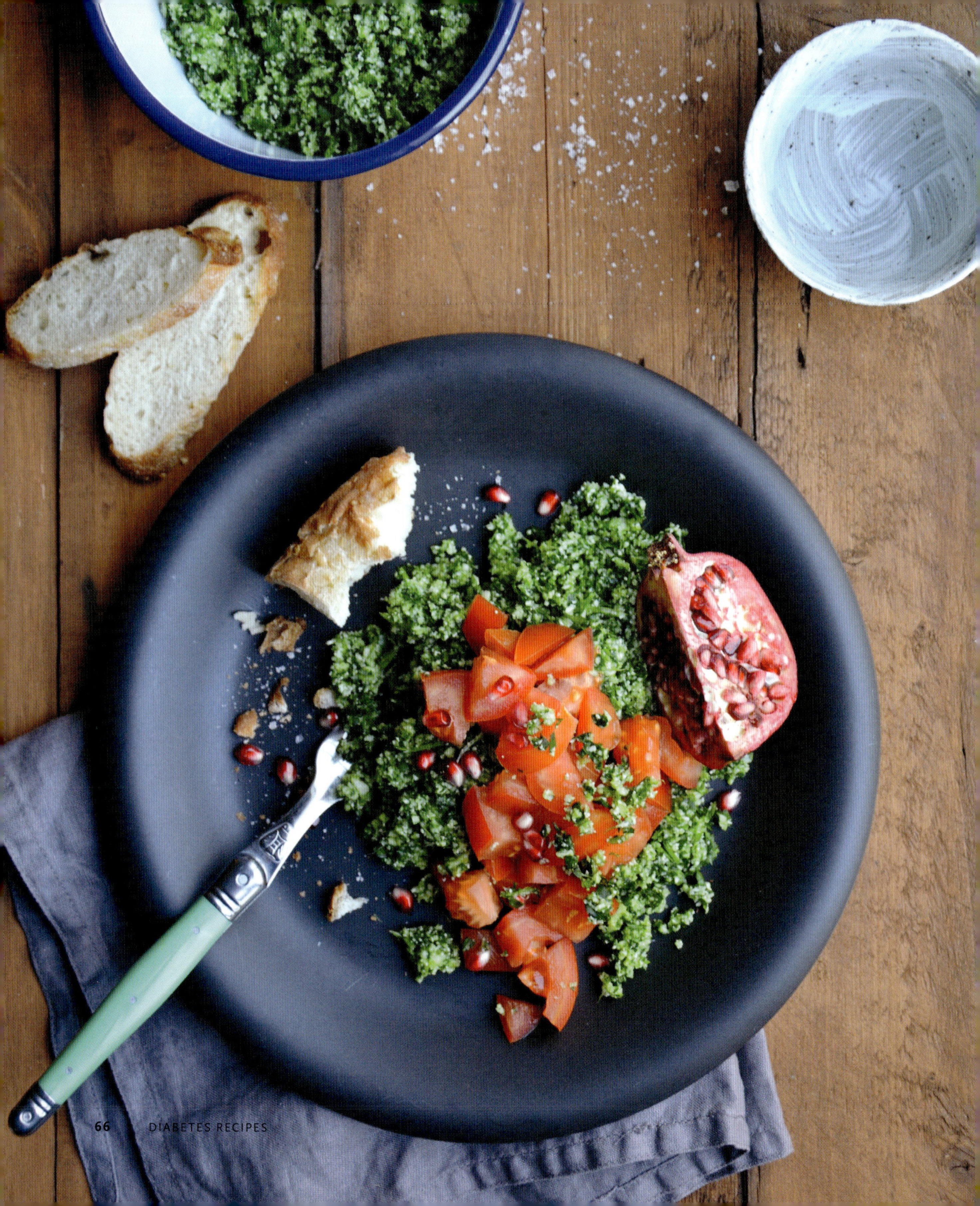

Cauliflower tabouli

A simple twist on a classic, this recipe replaces the burghul/bulgur (cracked wheat) usually found in tabouli with riced cauliflower. This is one dish that demonstrates the importance of setting your kitchen up with the best tools your budget allows. If a full-sized food processor is out of the question, start shopping around for a handheld processor; the bowl is generally smaller so you just make smaller batches.

SERVES 4

½ head of cauliflower
1 large bunch of parsley
1 cup (45g) coriander/cilantro
2 spring onions/scallions
Zest of 1 lemon
1 tbsp extra virgin olive oil
Pinch of sea salt and black pepper
½ cup (45g) pomegranate seeds (optional)

1 Remove the cauliflower leaves and chop the stalk and florets into chunks.

2 Using a food processor, pulse the cauliflower with the parsley and coriander until a fine crumb is formed.

3 Slice the spring onions finely and stir through the tabouli.

4 Add extra virgin olive oil, lemon zest, sea salt and black pepper to season.

5 Garnish with pomegranate seeds if using.

Cauliflower is a fibre-rich, non-starchy vegetable that can supply up to 50 per cent of your daily vitamin C dietary needs. It's incredibly versatile yet is often overlooked as a vegetable. It can be eaten raw, steamed, pureed or roasted.

Chilli pumpkin + goat cheese spread

You can substitute the pumpkin in this recipe with carrot or sweet potato for a similar taste and texture. You can also omit the butter and replace with 1 tbsp of hulled tahini to help add a depth of flavour to the steamed vegetable. When you compare the simple list of ingredients below to the ingredients list on the back of a tub of dip at the supermarket, you will discover how easy, satisfying and healthy making your own dips and spreads at home is, and all for a fraction of the cost of store-bought.

SERVES 2

200g/7 oz pumpkin (any variety)

1½ tbsp dried chilli flakes

½ tbsp unsalted butter

2 tbsp goat cheese

1 Remove the skin from the pumpkin and dice the flesh into even sized chunks. Steam the pumpkin for 5–6 minutes, either in a microwave or in a steamer basket on the stove top over a pot of simmering water.

2 Once the pumpkin is tender add the chilli flakes and butter. Use an immersion blender to blitz the mixture to a smooth consistency.

3 Add the goat cheese to a small bowl and stir vigorously until the cheese is a smooth paste.

4 Pour the pumpkin spread into a serving dish and gently stir through the goat cheese to create a marbled effect. Serve as a spread on fresh rye bread or as a dip for vegetable sticks.

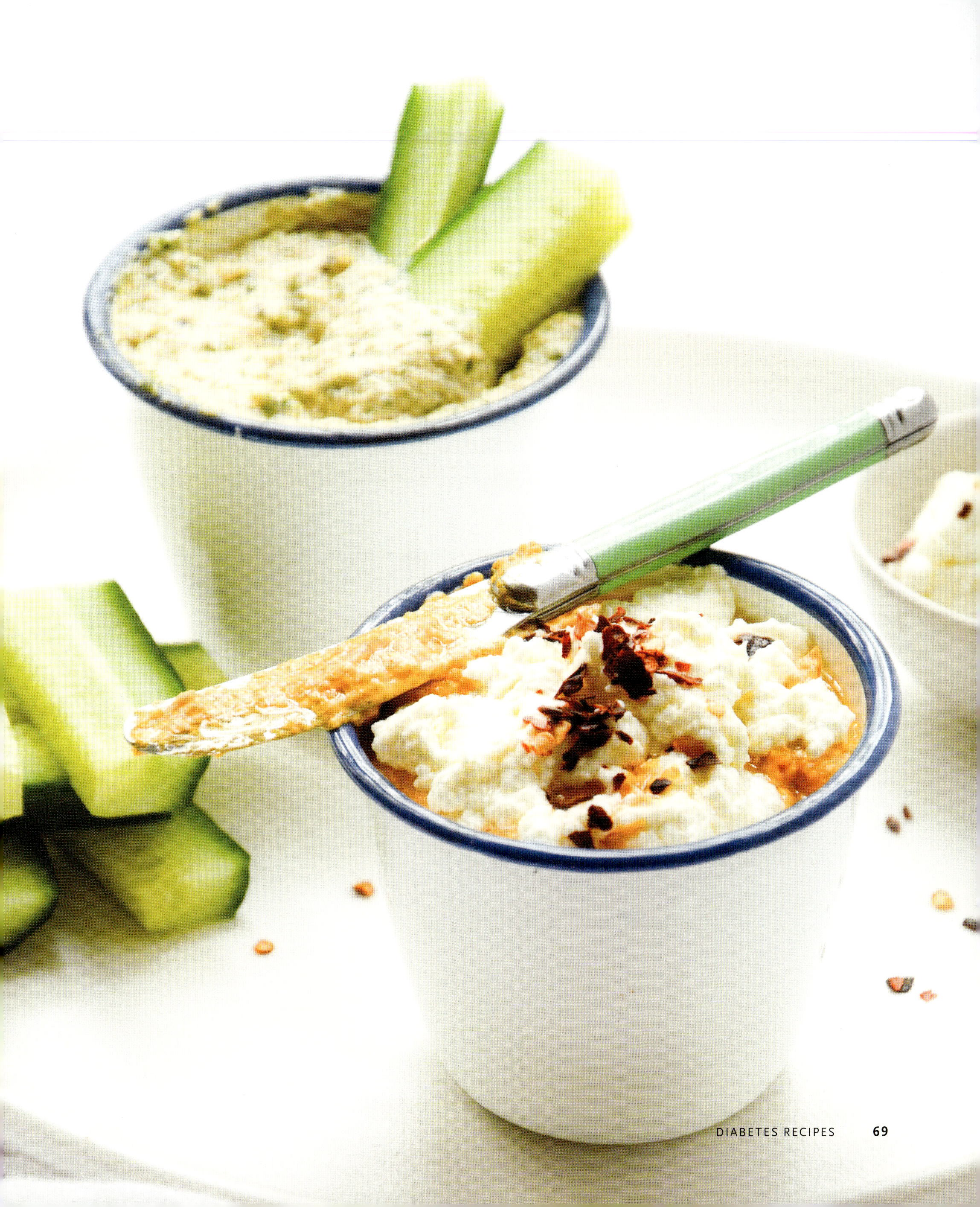

Zucchini hummus

SERVES 2

2 medium zucchinis/courgettes

Extra virgin olive oil

Pinch of sea salt and black pepper

2–3 heaped tbsp hulled tahini

¼ cup (10g) fresh dill

¼ cup (60ml) fresh lemon juice

1 Preheat the oven to 180°C/350°F.

2 Slice the zucchini in half lengthways, place on an oven tray lined with baking paper, drizzle a small amount of olive oil over the top and season with a pinch of sea salt and black pepper. Roast in the oven for 30 minutes until soft.

3 Place the zucchini, tahini, dill and lemon juice in the bowl of a food processor or use an immersion blender to mix into a smooth consistency. Store in the refrigerator for up to one week.

Lemon hummus

SERVES 2

200g/7 oz cooked chickpeas

1 tbsp hulled tahini

Juice and zest of ½ a lemon

¼–½ cup (60–125ml) extra virgin olive oil or water

Sea salt and black pepper

Add the chickpeas, tahini, lemon juice and zest to the bowl of a food processor with the feed tube open. Pour in a little olive oil at a time as you mix on medium speed. The amount of oil added will depend on the consistency you want the hummus. Blend until smooth, taste then season with sea salt and black pepper. You could also add a garlic clove to the mixture or spices such as smoked paprika or cumin.

Avocado white bean smash

SERVES 2

1 medium avocado

½ cup (100g) cooked cannellini beans (or other white bean)

¼ cup (60ml) fresh lemon juice

¼ cup (10g) flat leaf parsley, finely chopped

1 tsp chilli flakes (or fresh chilli)

1 tsp sea salt

In a mixing bowl combine the avocado flesh, cannellini beans, lemon juice, parsley, chilli and salt. Use the back of a fork to roughly mash the ingredients together. You can use an immersion blender to do this but I like to keep some texture to the dish and a fork does this easily. Serve on toasted rye bread or as a dip for fresh vegetables.

Baba ganoush dip

SERVES 2

2 large eggplants/aubergines

Extra virgin olive oil

3 tsp sea salt

1 tbp smoked paprika

1 tsp ground cumin

2 garlic cloves

2 tbsp hulled tahini

1 Preheat the oven to 180°C/350°F.

2 Prick each eggplant several times with a fork, knife or skewer. Using a gas burner, BBQ hotplate or a grill/broiler, char the skin of the eggplants for 5 minutes to help create a smoky flavour.

3 Transfer the eggplants to a baking dish or oven tray, drizzle the olive oil over the top and sprinkle over the sea salt, smoked paprika and cumin. Add the garlic cloves to the tray and roast for 30 minutes or until soft and caramelised.

4 Peel the charred skin and add the eggplant flesh and the garlic to the bowl of a food processor and blitz with the tahini until smooth.

Basic sauerkraut

MAKES 1 MEDIUM JAR

¼–½ head savoy cabbage

2 tbsp sea salt flakes

1 tsp caraway seeds

1 Remove the core from the cabbage, reserve 1 or 2 outer leaves to the side and finely slice the rest of the leaves. Add the cabbage to a large bowl with the salt and caraway seeds and massage with your hands for 5 minutes. As you work the salt into the leaves you will notice liquid forming at the bottom of the bowl, keep massaging until the cabbage has softened and is damp.

2 Sterilise a medium sized glass jar in boiling water then stuff the cabbage firmly into the jar, pushing down to compact it as much as possible, leaving a good couple of inches at the top of the jar. Fold the reserved cabbage leaves in half and stuff into the top of the jar to weigh the sauerkraut down.

3 At this stage you can place a piece of muslin cloth over the top of the jar, loosely place the jar lid on top, or secure the jar lid. Store the sauerkraut on your kitchen bench for three days before moving it to the fridge. If you have secured a lid on the jar, open the jar every day while it's on the bench to release the gas forming.

4 The sauerkraut can be enjoyed on top of scrambled eggs for breakfast, in salads, or simply a forkful at a time. Be careful not to double dip, rather remove a portion from the jar then eat, instead of returning the fork into the kraut again and again, this will help avoid contamination and early spoilage.

Fermenting fresh vegetables, such as the humble cabbage, is a great way to provide beneficial probiotics to your gut as well as delivering a tasty addition to your plate. Basic fermenting at home is easy, and once you're confident with sauerkraut and kim chi you can begin experimenting with more complicated recipes. When starting out, aim to make smaller batches as you hone your skills and discover what tastes you like.

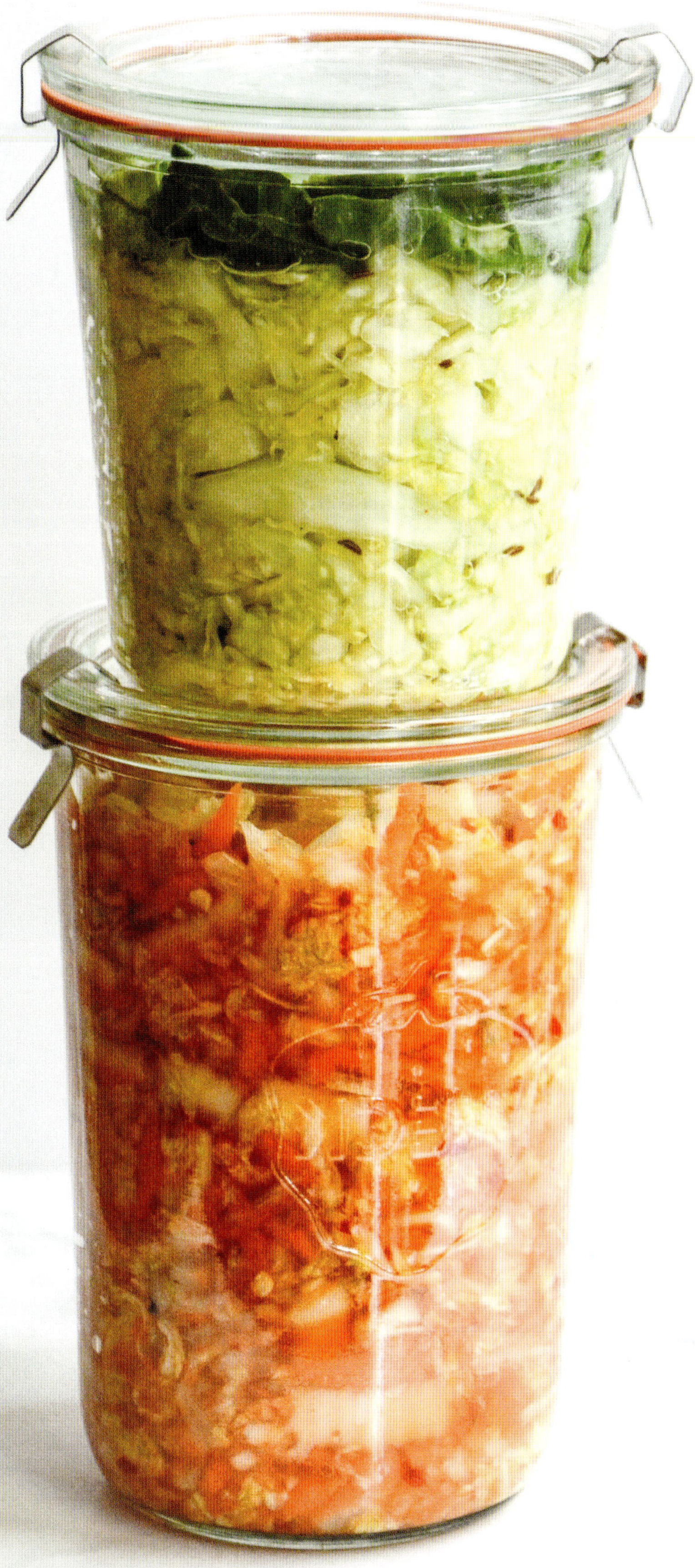

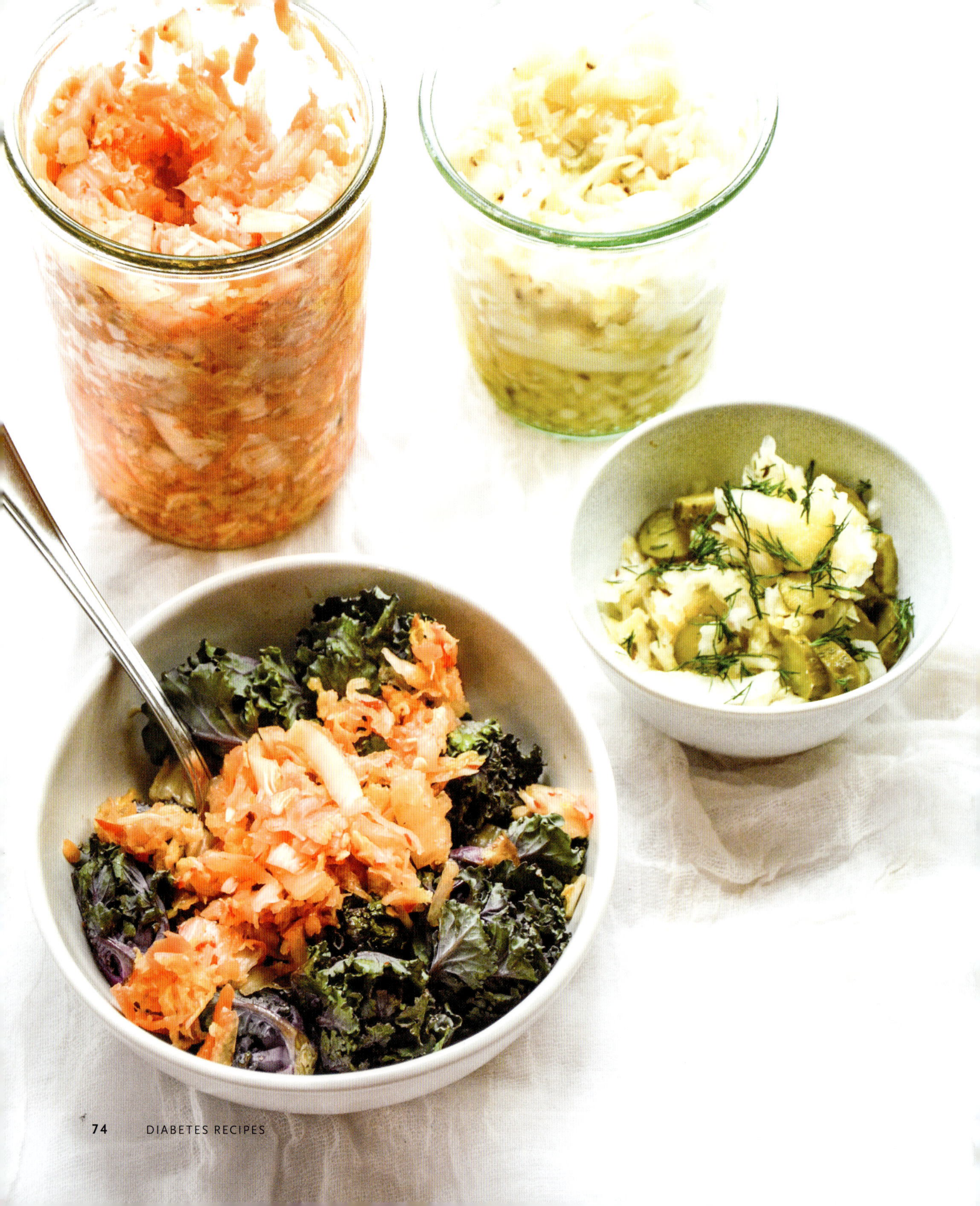

Simple kim chi

MAKES 1 LARGE JAR

1 large wombok/Chinese cabbage or white cabbage

¼ cup (20g) sea salt

Filtered water

4 garlic cloves

1 inch piece of ginger

4 long red chillis

2 tbsp water

1 large daikon/radish

2 large carrots

3 spring onions/scallions

1 Remove the core from the cabbage and slice the remaining leaves, either finely or into medium sized chunks. Add the cabbage and salt to a large bowl and massage with your hands to soften the leaves. Pour enough water into the bowl to just cover the cabbage and weigh it down with a plate. At this stage you can leave the cabbage to rest anywhere from 1 hour to overnight.

2 Rinse the cabbage in fresh filtered water to remove the excess salt then thoroughly drain the cabbage. Wash the soaking bowl then add the cabbage back in.

3 Add the garlic, ginger, chilli and water to the bowl of a food processor and blitz into a paste, adding more water if necessary.

4 Finely chop or shred the daikon, carrots and spring onion and add to the bowl of cabbage. At this stage you may want to wear rubber or disposable gloves as you add the chilli mixture to the cabbage and work it through the vegetables.

5 Sterilise a large glass jar with boiling water then stuff the kim chi mix into it, pushing down hard to compact it. There should be a small amount of liquid covering the top of the kim chi at this point. Seal the jar and leave it to ferment on the kitchen counter for 3–5 days before storing it in the fridge for a further week before eating. The flavour will intensify the longer it is left so taste it after a week to see if it's to your liking or if it needs more time.

Eat kim chi with a bowl of fresh greens or try sauerkraut with dill + pickled cucumber.

Peach, prosciutto + goat cheese rolls

This is a classic pairing of sweet and savoury and is a quick and easy snack to prepare for yourself or as a party appetiser. You can omit the goat cheese for a dairy free option.

MAKES 6

1 large peach, any variety

1 tbsp maple syrup (optional)

1 tsp vanilla powder

6 thin slices of prosciutto or ham

6 tsp smooth goat cheese

6 skewers

1 Preheat the oven to 180°C/350°F. Cut the peach in half, remove the stone and cut each half into thirds. Place the peach pieces into an oven tray and drizzle over the maple syrup (if using) and vanilla powder. Roast in the oven for 15 minutes until soft but still holding its shape. Remove from the oven and set aside to cool.

2 Lay the prosciutto or ham slices on a board and spread the goat cheese in a thin layer from one end of each to the other. Take the cooled peaches and place one at the edge of each slice of prosciutto. Roll the prosciutto over the peach until covered then place a skewer through the middle to hold it in place.

3 Store in the fridge until ready to serve.

Wedges of crisp apple or pear also taste great when rolled in proscuitto, with or without the goat cheese. Sprinkle ground cinnamon on the apple before rolling for a spicy flavour boost.

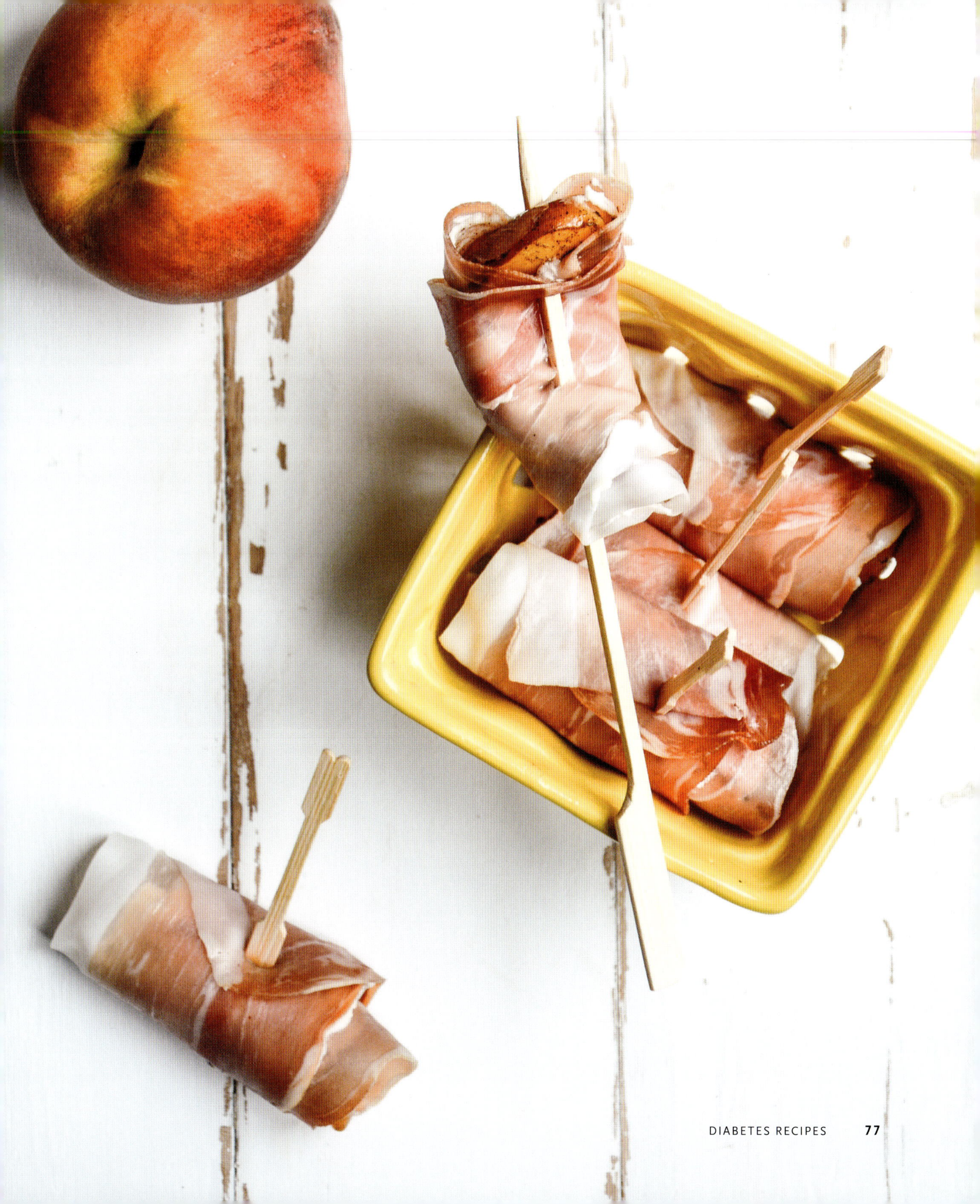

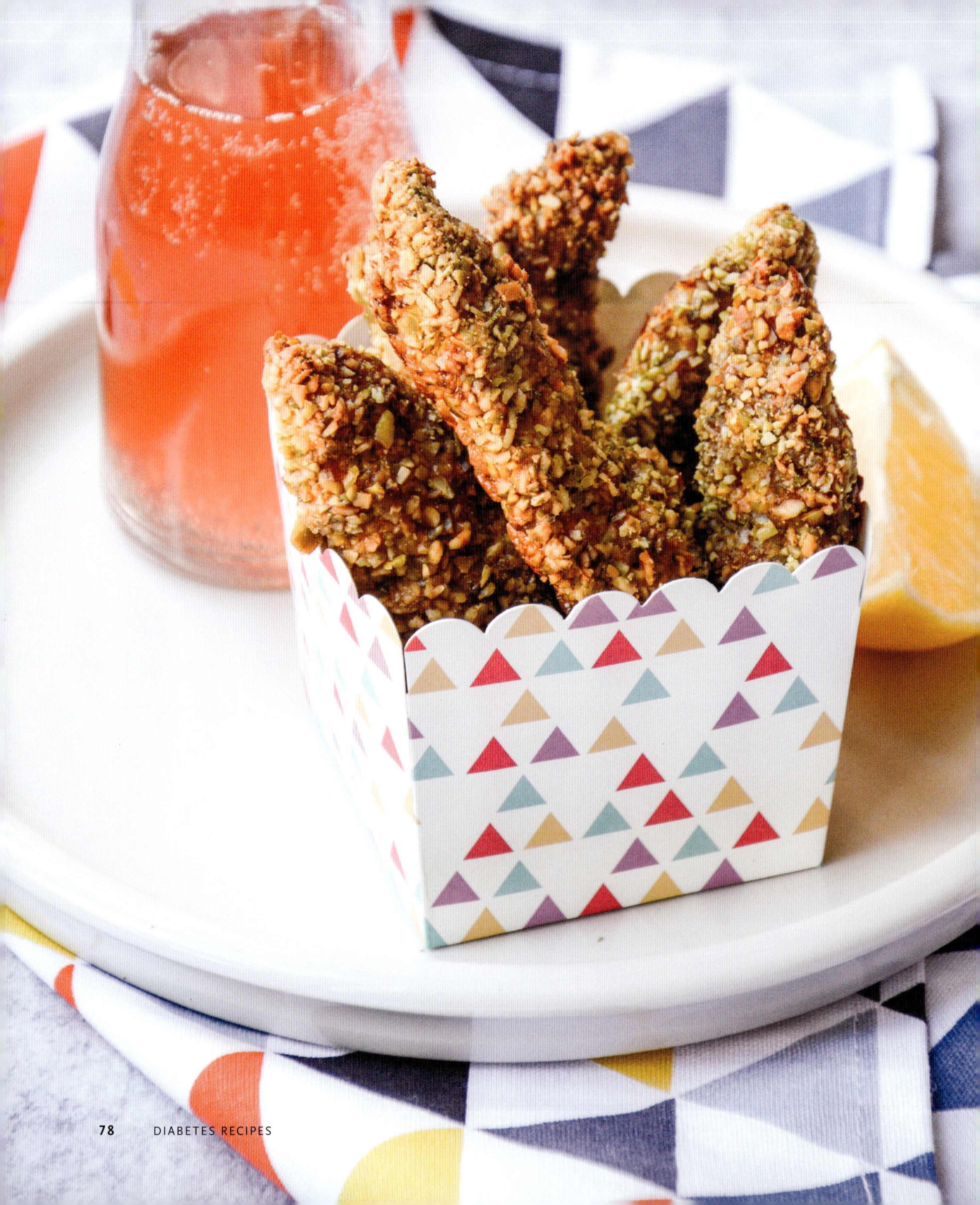

Pepita crusted chicken strips

These baked chicken strips are coated in pumpkin seeds rather than the usual breadcrumb coating found on schnitzels or other types of crumbed chicken. Pumpkin seeds offer a great amount of antioxidants and are high in zinc, magnesium and potassium. You can make these chicken strips ahead of time and freeze either cooked or raw.

MAKES 12

400g/14 oz chicken breast fillets

1 cup (140g) pepitas/pumpkin seeds

1 cup (125g) brown rice flour

2 free range eggs

Sea salt

Optional extras: ¼ cup (20g) grated Parmesan cheese, 2 tbsp dried basil

1 Preheat the oven to 180°C/350°F.

2 Using a food processor fitted with the S blade attachment, or using a handheld immersion blender, blitz the pepitas until crushed. Spread out over a plate.

3 On another plate sprinkle the flour. If using the additional seasonings, add to the flour and stir through.

4 Crack the eggs into a bowl and whisk with a fork until just combined.

5 Slice the chicken breast fillets into strips. Dip each strip into the flour followed by the egg and finally coat in the crushed pepitas. Place each strip on an oven tray lined with baking paper before sprinkling a pinch of sea salt over the top. Bake for 20–30 minutes, testing one strip to check the chicken is cooked through before removing them all.

These make great party food for adults and kids alike. Serve with wedges of fresh lemon.

Potato wedges with guacamole

Baking these wedges instead of shallow or deep frying makes them a healthier snack option while still delivering a great taste. Serve with guacamole for dipping the wedges into rather than tomato or sweet chilli sauce, which can be loaded with refined sugar.

SERVES 2

2 potatoes, any variety

½ tbsp extra virgin olive oil

Sea salt and smoked paprika for seasoning

GUACAMOLE

1 avocado

Juice and zest of 1 lemon

Pinch of sea salt and black pepper

Fresh chives for garnish

1 Preheat the oven to its highest setting.

2 Slice the potatoes into even, chip-shaped chunks. Bring 2 cups (500ml) of water to a simmer in a saucepan then place the potatoes in a steamer basket or colander over the top and cover with the saucepan lid. Steam the potatoes for 10 minutes until a knife easily goes through.

3 Place the potatoes in a bowl and pour over the oil, toss gently. Spread the potatoes evenly over an oven tray (line with baking paper if needed) and bake for 25 minutes, turning frequently until crisp. It can be easier to use an egg flip or spatula to slide under the wedges and turn, rather than using tongs. Remove the wedges from the oven and season with sea salt and smoked paprika if desired.

4 To prepare the guacamole, add the avocado flesh, lemon juice and zest, and sea salt and black pepper to the bowl of a food processor and blitz to desired consistency. Alternatively you can mash the avocado using a fork. Garnish the guacamole with finely chopped chives.

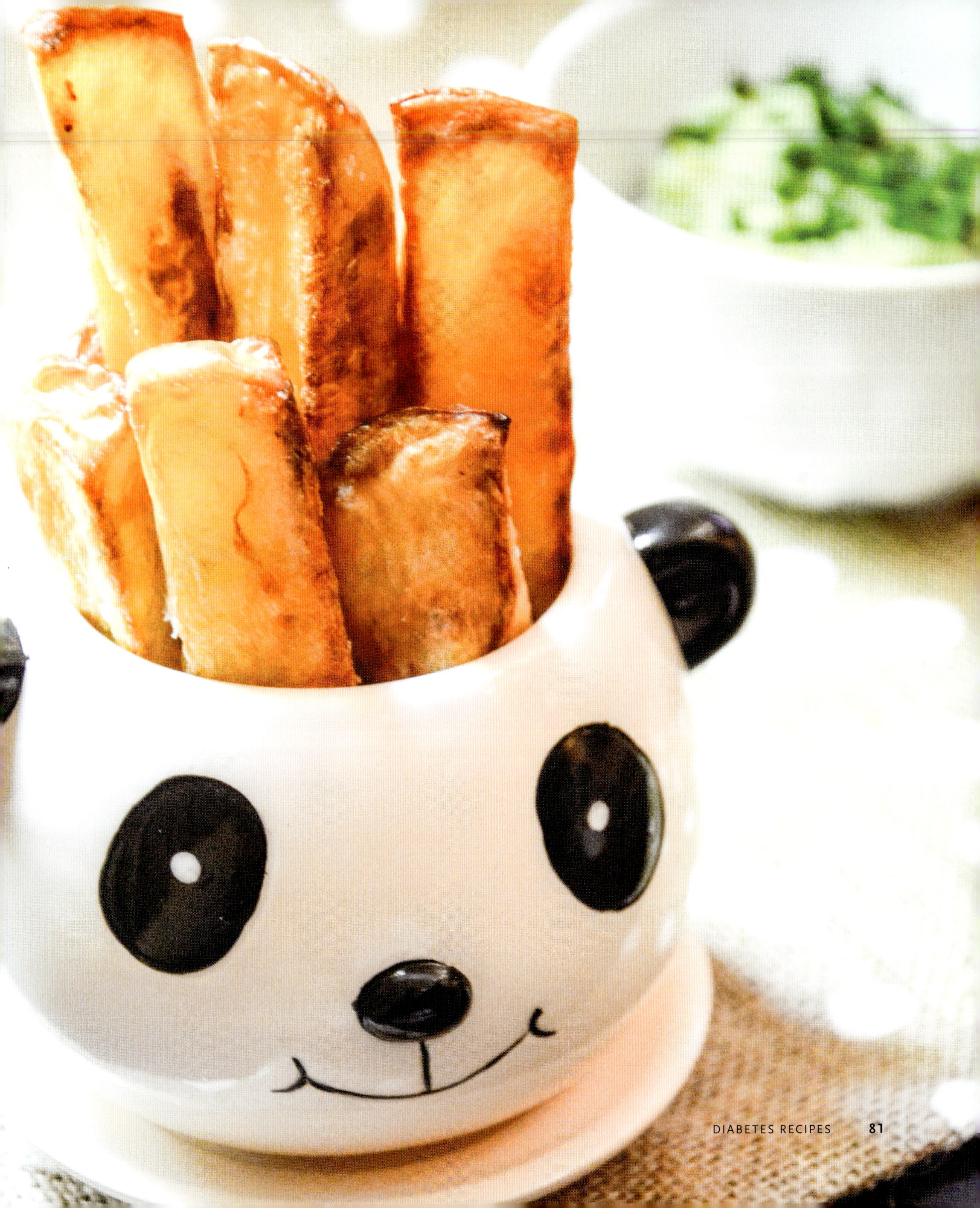

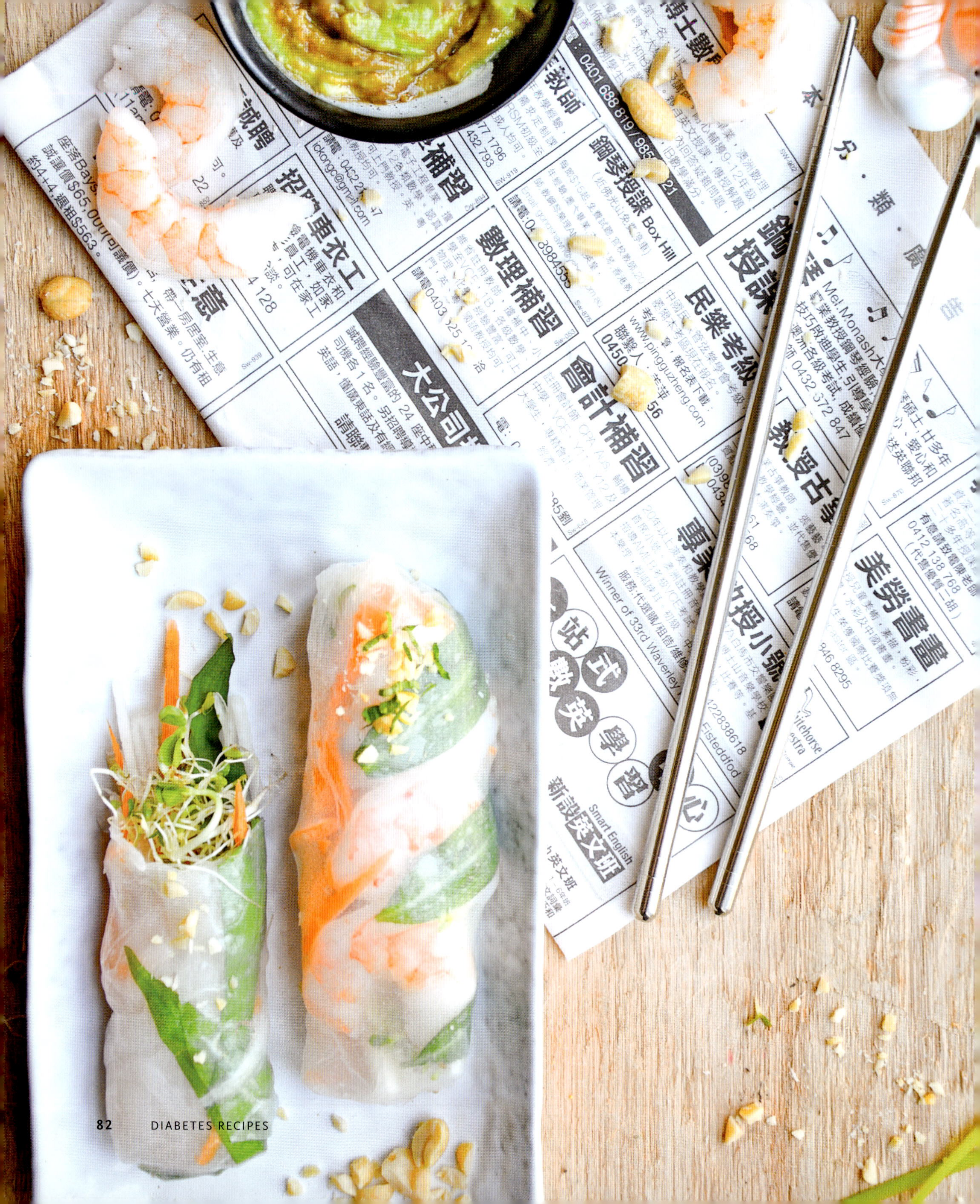

Prawn + sprouts rice paper rolls

Make these ahead of time for an easy grab-and-go lunch or snack. Substitute the prawns for cooked strips of chicken or beef, or keep it vegetarian and stuff the rolls full of finely sliced or shredded vegetables and leaves.

MAKES 6

12 cooked prawns, any variety

1 large carrot

½ daikon (white radish)

6 rice paper sheets

1 cup (30g) snow pea or alfalfa sprouts

12 Thai basil leaves

DIPPING SAUCE

½ an avocado

Juice of ½ a lemon

2 tbsp Tamari/wheat free soy sauce

½ cup (75g) unsalted cashews or other nut (optional)

1 Prep the prawns by removing the tails and making sure they are clean. Set aside. Julienne the carrot and daikon using a peeler or finely slicing with a knife. Set aside.

2 Fill a large bowl with warm water and hydrate the rice paper sheets one at a time following packet instructions. Place the hydrated rice paper sheet on a damp tea towel and begin adding the fillings on one side of the sheet, starting with the sprouts and basil leaves and layering prawns, carrot and daikon (use two prawns per rice paper roll). Fold the sides in and roll the rice paper sheet up, securing with a dab of water if needed.

3 Prepare the dipping sauce by blitzing the avocado and lemon juice in a food processor or by using an immersion blender. Stir through the Tamari, starting with 1 tbsp and adding more according to desired taste. Roughly chop the cashews and place in a bowl next to the dipping sauce.

mains

Lemon lentil soup
Cauliflower + horseradish soup
Beef bone broth
Spicy beef + Tuscan kale stew
Potato + snow pea green curry
Quinoa "fried rice"
Herbed mushrooms on socca
Sweet potato, black bean + jalapeño burger patties
Pulled cider pork with roasted garlic + apple salad
Chicken + avocado skewers
Sweet potato noodle stir-fry
Roast paprika chicken
Dukkah crusted chicken maryland with confetti rice
Cashew satay beef skewers
Meatball subs with tomato relish
Instant noodle pots
Pan seared salmon with dill pea mash
Veg packed bolognaise

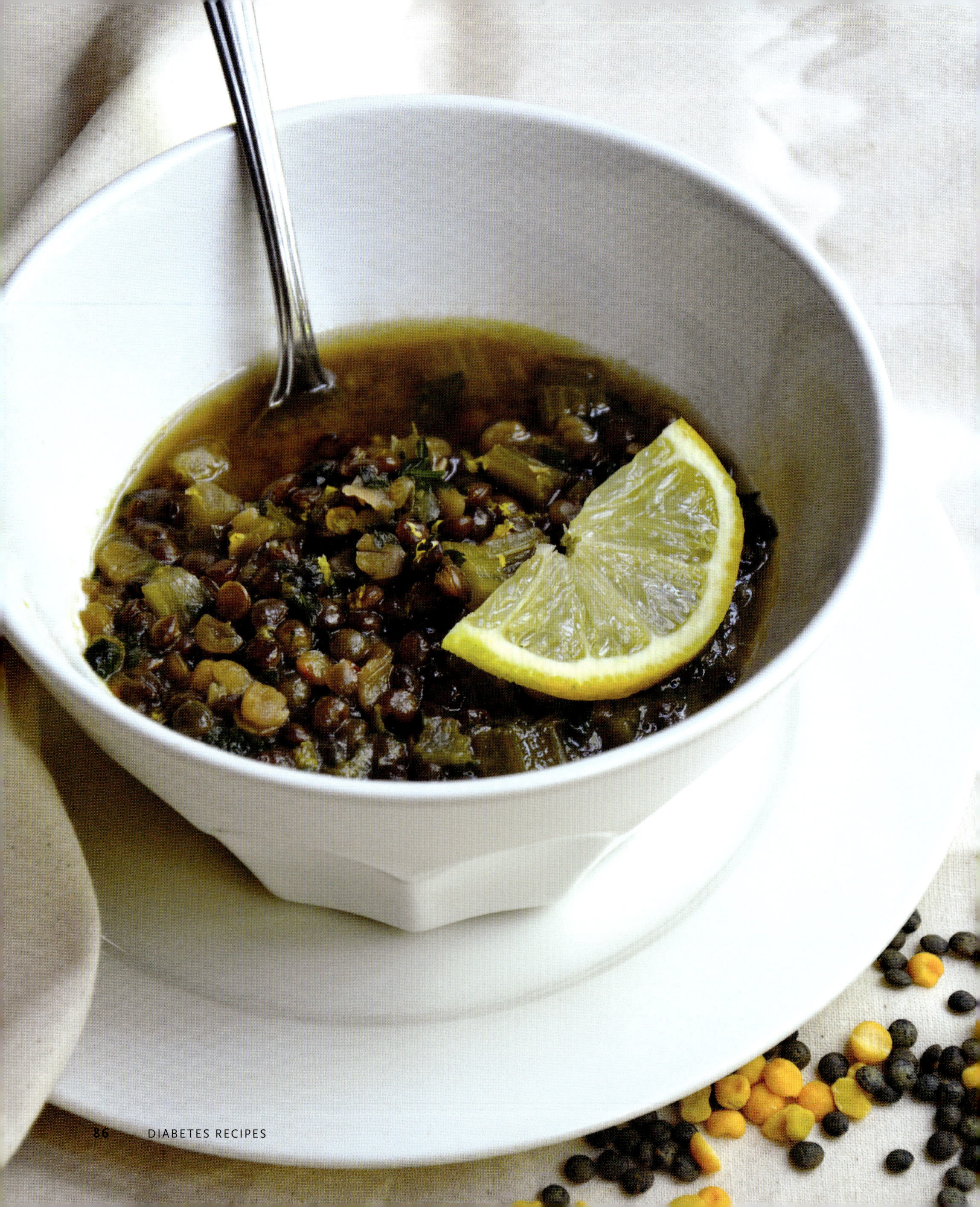

Lemon lentil soup

Soup is often thought of as a warming winter meal, and while this lentil soup is delicious when it's cold outside, the addition of zingy lemon and fresh parsley makes it a wonderful meal in other seasons also. Make your own stock and freeze it in ice cube trays for easy access when you need it, or use a good quality store-bought stock that's low in sodium and free of additives or preservatives. Add extra vegetables to the soup to customise to your tastes, or use additional herbs such as thyme for added depth of flavour.

SERVES 4

4 celery stalks, thinly sliced

4 cups (1L) chicken or vegetable stock

1 cup (200g) dried lentils (any variety)

Zest and juice of ½ a lemon

Sea salt and black pepper

½ cup (25g) parsley, finely chopped

1 Soften the celery stalks in a stock pot with a drizzle of olive oil.

2 Add the chicken or vegetable stock followed by the lentils.

3 Cook for 30 minutes, stirring occasionally.

4 Remove the soup from the heat and stir in the lemon zest, lemon juice, salt, pepper and parsley.

Unlike beans, lentils don't necessarily need to be soaked before cooking. It can, however, help with digestion to rinse the lentils and soak in a bowl of filtered water for one hour. Rinse the lentils again before cooking.

Cauliflower + horseradish soup

This creamy soup has a delicious bite thanks to the addition of horseradish. It can be hard to source fresh horseradish so if you can't find any, substitute with a good quality horseradish cream, taking time to read the ingredients list and choosing the brand with no added sugar and preferably no seed oils. You could also substitute the horseradish for fresh chilli or wasabi, which will give you a different sort of heat but will still compliment the soup nicely.

SERVES 4

1 head of cauliflower

2 parsnips or potatoes, cleaned but not peeled

25g/1 oz butter

8 cups (2L) vegetable stock plus additional water as needed

3 tbsp fresh horseradish, grated

Sea salt and black pepper

1 bunch of fresh chives

1 Remove the florets from the cauliflower and dice the stalk into small chunks.

2 Clean the parsnip, discard the ends and dice into even chunks.

3 Add the cauliflower, parsnip and butter to a large stockpot and sweat for 10 minutes with a pinch of sea salt before adding the vegetable stock and cooking over a medium heat for 40 minutes or until the vegetables are tender.

4 Add the horseradish to the soup then puree the mixture using an immersion blender, making sure there are no chunks of vegetables left. If the soup is too thick, add a dash of water at a time until you reach the desired consistency. Taste the soup and season with salt and pepper if needed.

5 Chop the chives and scatter over the soup before serving.

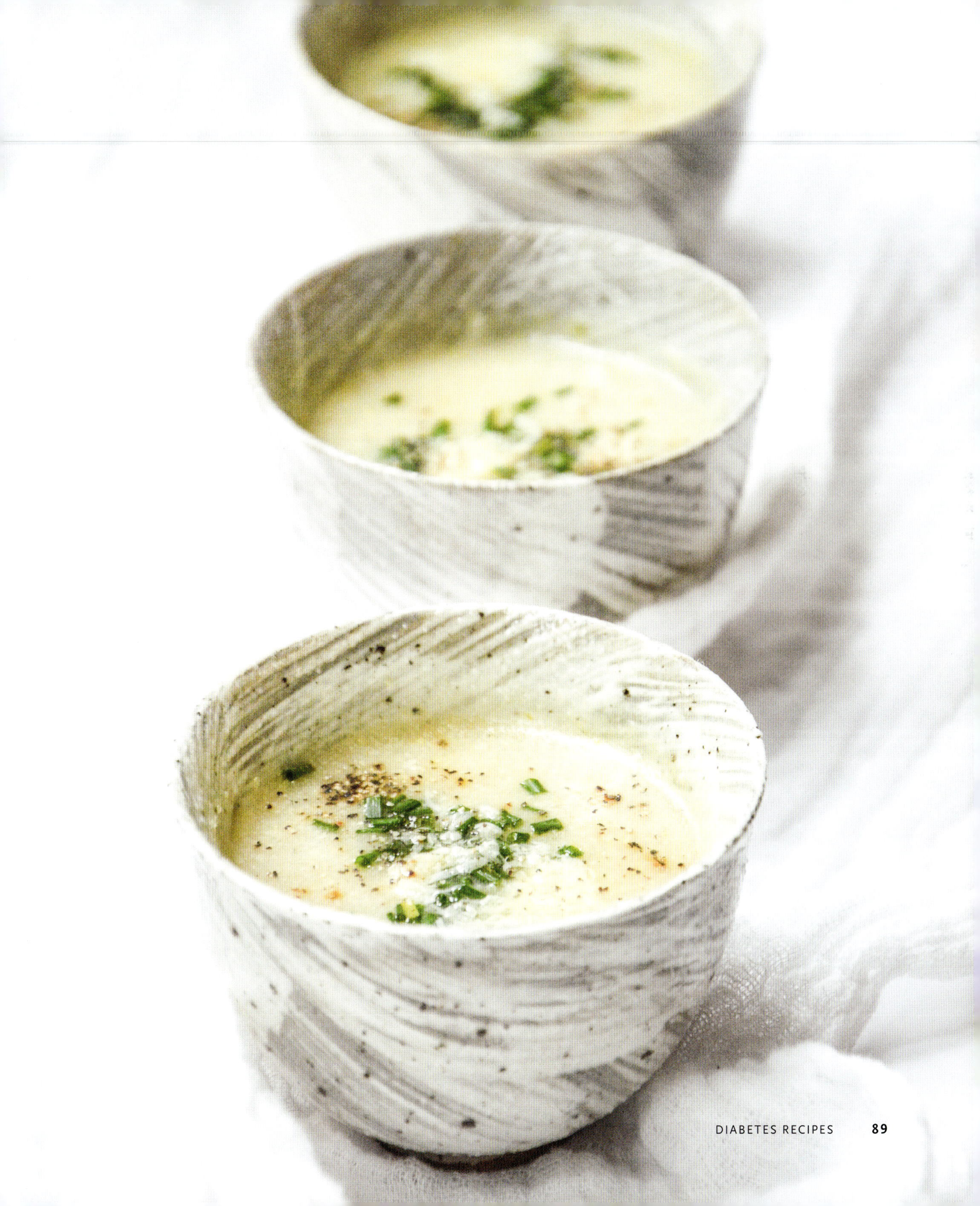

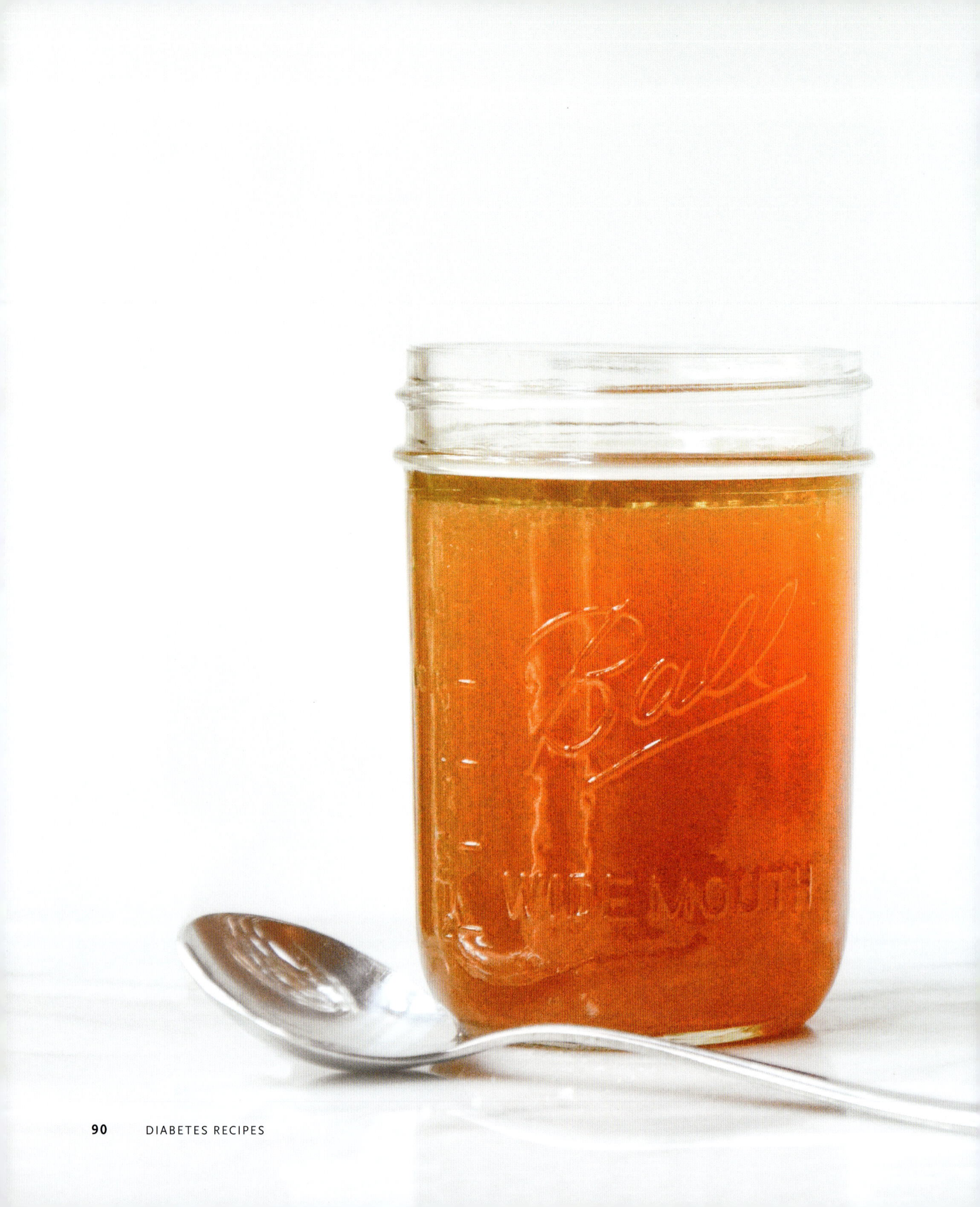
Ball
WIDE MOUTH

Beef bone broth

Bone broth is a great addition to your daily diet for a number of reasons. Firstly, it's extremely economical to make; it's also incredibly easy, it's just a matter of adding everything to the pot and leaving it to simmer and bubble away for hours on end. Bone broth is packed full of minerals that we often miss out on in diets that are more centred on fillets of meat and not the whole animal. Studies suggest that including bone broth in your diet helps you better absorb other proteins, and the gelatine extracted from the bones is great for your joints, skin and hair. By freezing the broth in ice cube trays, you can pop a couple of cubes out at a time and heat them up for a warming drink when you don't want to use the broth for a soup or stew.

1.5kg/3 lb grass fed beef bones

¼ cup (60ml) apple cider vinegar

Enough filtered water to cover the bones

1 large brown onion

2 carrots

4 celery stalks, including leaves

1 star anise

6 peppercorns

Stalks from 1 bunch of parsley

1 Preheat the oven to 180°C/350°F.

2 Place the beef bones in a large stockpot with the apple cider vinegar and let it sit for half an hour.

3 Add the onion, carrots and celery then place the pot over a medium heat and add enough filtered water to cover the bones and vegetables. Add the star anise, peppercorns and parsley stalks, bring the mixture to the boil then reduce the heat to low.

4 Cook the broth on low for at least 8 hours, topping up the liquid in the pot with additional water as needed so the bones are consistently covered. If you have a slow cooker you can cook the broth on low overnight, which will help draw out even more minerals and collagen. It's easy to set the slow cooker for 8 hours during the day then follow it up with 8 hours overnight, which will give you premium bone broth with minimal effort.

5 When ready, strain the bones, vegetables, star anise and peppercorns from the liquid. Store some broth in a jar in the refrigerator to be consumed within 24 hours. If you're not immediately using the rest for a soup or stew then pour any remaining broth into freezer-friendly containers or ice cube trays for later use.

Spicy beef + Tuscan kale stew

This warming stew is simply a matter of throwing everything in the pot and giving it time. Keeping the ingredients list short allows each flavour to truly shine. Adjust the spiciness of the dish to suit your taste or omit the chillis entirely for a milder dish. You can add extra vegetables beyond the kale and pumpkin, stir through a tin of chickpeas or serve on a bed of mashed potato.

SERVES 2–4

500g/1 lb sirloin or rump steak

½ Spanish/red onion, finely chopped

1 inch piece of fresh ginger root, finely grated

4 garlic cloves, crushed

2–3 red chillis (any variety), finely chopped

1 cup (250g) diced tomatoes

2 cups (500ml) beef broth (page 91), plus more stock or water as needed

300g/10.5 oz pumpkin, any variety

1 bunch of Tuscan kale

1 Slice the beef into thin strips or cut into chunks and sprinkle lightly with sea salt.

2 Heat up a large cast iron pot or saucepan over a medium heat. Add a drizzle of extra virgin olive oil and add the onion, ginger, garlic and chilli. Sweat for 3–5 minutes.

3 Add the beef, tomatoes and stock, stir and reduce the heat to low.

4 Cut the pumpkin into chunks and add to the pot. Simmer for 35 minutes until the beef is tender, checking every 15 minutes and adding additional stock or water as needed.

5 Remove the stem from the Tuscan kale and cut the leaves into medium sized chunks. Add the kale to the stew and cook for 20 minutes before serving.

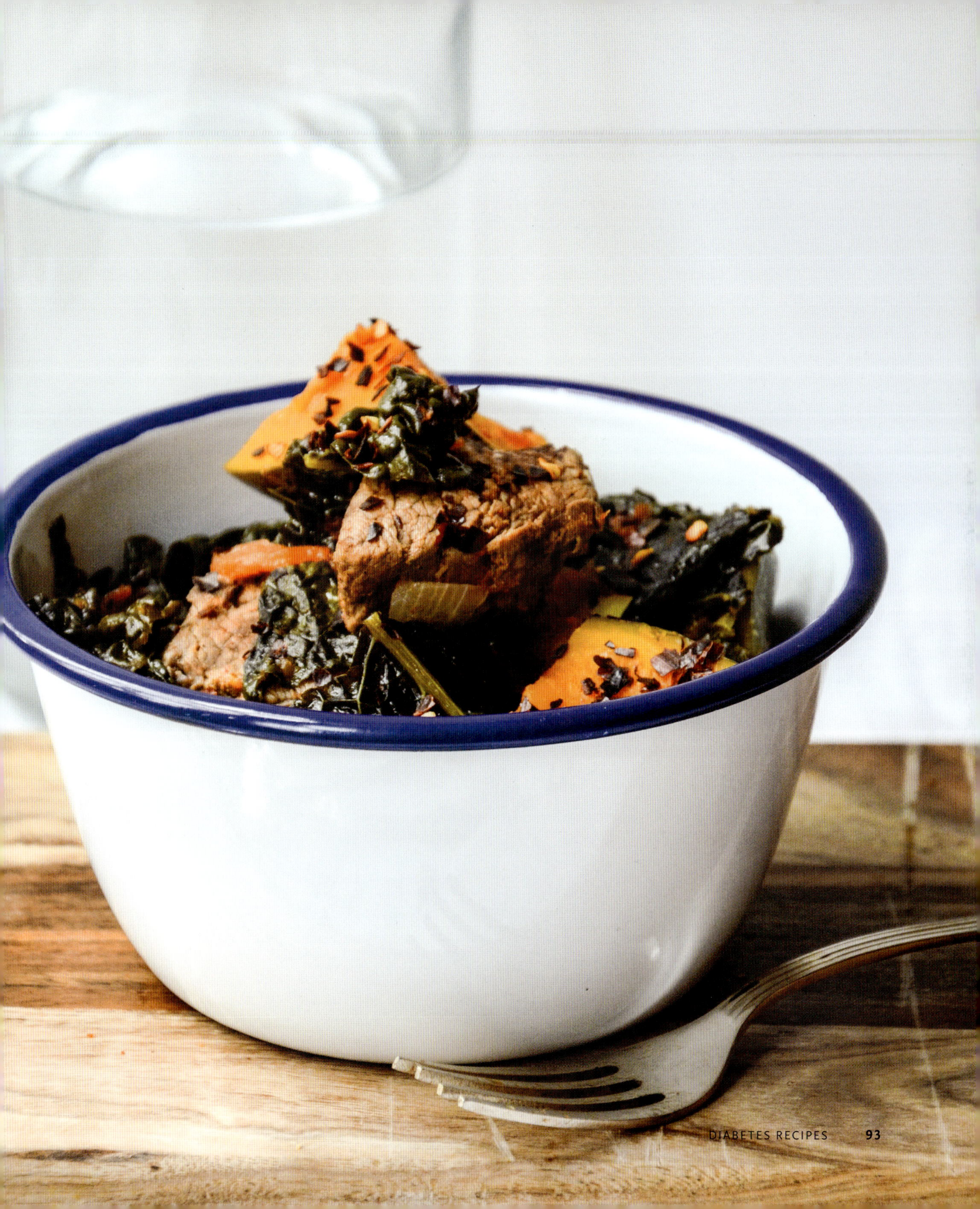

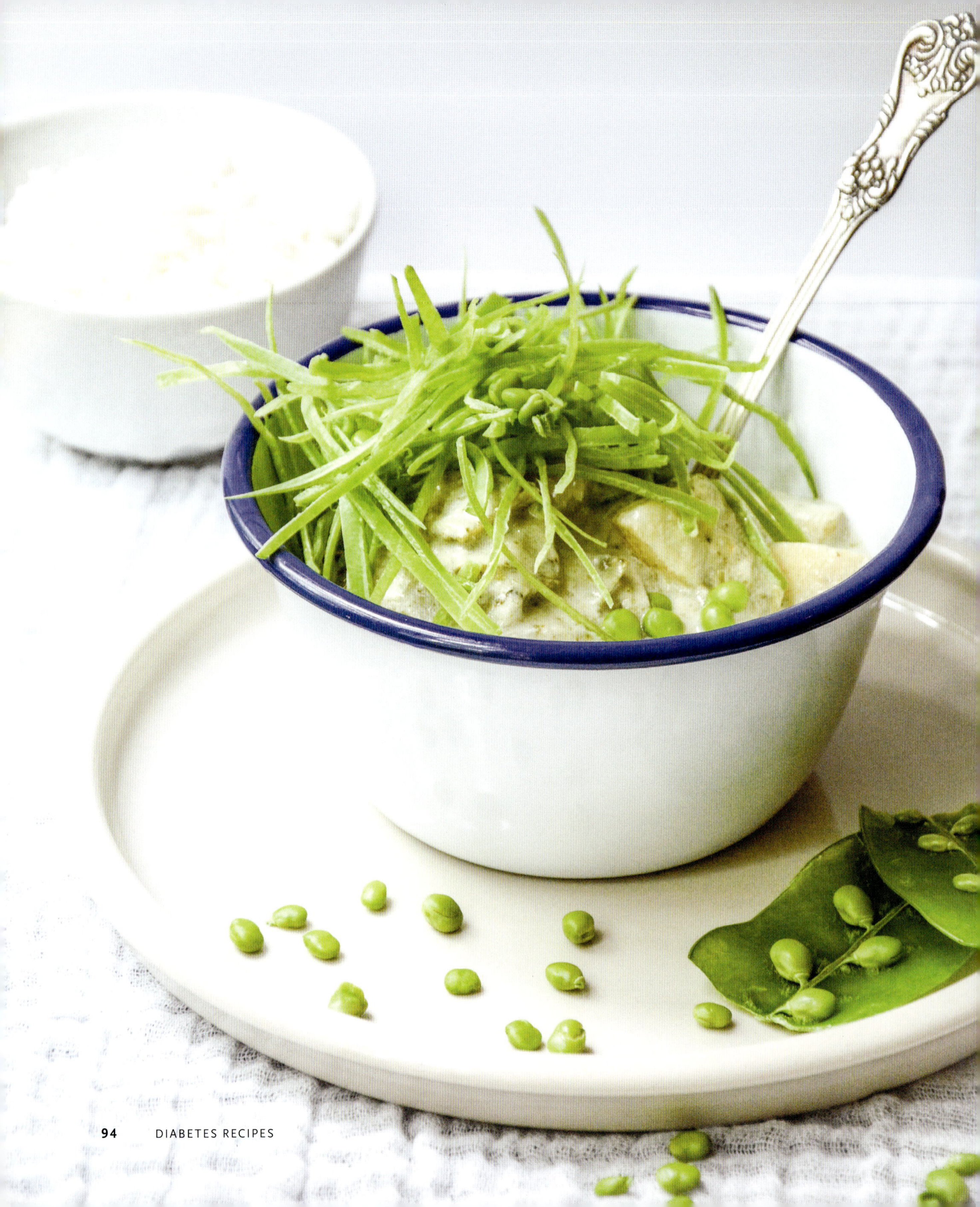

Potato + snow pea green curry

Making a curry paste at home is incredibly simple with the help of a food processor to blitz everything together for you but you can also use a mortar and pestle along with a little elbow grease. Make the paste ahead of time, such as on the weekend, store in an airtight jar or container in the fridge and you'll have it ready to go for a mid-week meal. You can mix up the ingredients by replacing the potato with pumpkin, sweet potato or cauliflower, or add chicken and beef if you're not going meat free.

SERVES 4

CURRY PASTE

1 lemongrass stalk

1 inch chunk of galangal

1 inch chunk of fresh ginger

Handful of fresh Thai basil leaves

2–4 green chillis (depending on desired heat)

4 garlic cloves

2 shallots

2 coriander/cilantro roots, washed

1 tbsp ground coriander

1 tbsp ground cumin

⅓ cup (80ml) olive oil, plus more as needed

Pinch of sea salt

8 medium potatoes

2 cups (500ml) coconut milk

300g/10.5 oz snow peas, trimmed

1 cup (250ml) filtered water, plus more as needed

Corinader/ cilantro for serving (optional)

1 Prepare the curry paste by removing the outer leaves of the lemongrass and cutting the stalk into chunks. Add the lemongrass to the bowl of a food processor or blender along with the galangal, ginger, basil leaves, chillis, garlic, shallots, coriander root, ground coriander, cumin, olive oil and sea salt. Blitz until a paste forms, stopping every now and then to scrape down the sides of the bowl and add a touch more oil for lubrication if needed.

2 Heat a large pot on medium on the stove then add the curry paste and cook until it becomes fragrant, for 3–5 minutes. Pour in the coconut milk and stir to remove any stuck on bits on the bottom of the pan.

3 Dice the potatoes, skin on, into even chunks and add to the pan of sauce. Stir to coat the potatoes then reduce the heat to low, cover the pot with a lid and let the curry simmer for 45 minutes, checking occasionally and adding a dash of water if the mixture is drying up.

4 Top and tail the snow peas and add whole or sliced into strips to the curry once the potatoes are tender. Stir through, taste and season with additional sea salt or black pepper if needed. Cook for a further 15 minutes before removing from the heat so as not to overcook the snow peas.

5 Serve the curry with rice, quinoa or on its own, topped with fresh coriander if using.

Quinoa "fried rice"

Swap the old-school fried rice with soy sauce and shrimp for a lighter, healthier version using quinoa. This is a great recipe to make using leftover quinoa, or simply cook some for this dish. Add whatever vegetables you have on hand in the fridge or stick to the classic scrambled egg, peas, capsicum and spring onion.

SERVES 4

3 free range eggs

1 red capsicum/pepper

1 cup (120g) cooked peas

3 spring onions/scallions

2 celery stalks

Handful of coriander/cilantro leaves

2 cups (370g) cooked quinoa

Juice of 1 lemon

Sea salt and black pepper

1 Crack the eggs into a bowl and whisk with a fork. Heat up a small frying pan and scramble the egg until cooked to your liking. Set aside.

2 Dice the red capsicum, finely slice the spring onions and celery stalks and add to a bowl. Finely chop the coriander leaves and add to the bowl.

3 Add the cooked quinoa to the bowl followed by the lemon juice and a pinch of sea salt and black pepper. Stir through the scrambled egg until all the ingredients are combined.

Serve this "fried rice" alongside a piece of grilled steak or chicken, enjoy it as a salad on its own or even as an easy breakfast with a fried egg on top instead of scrambled into the mix.

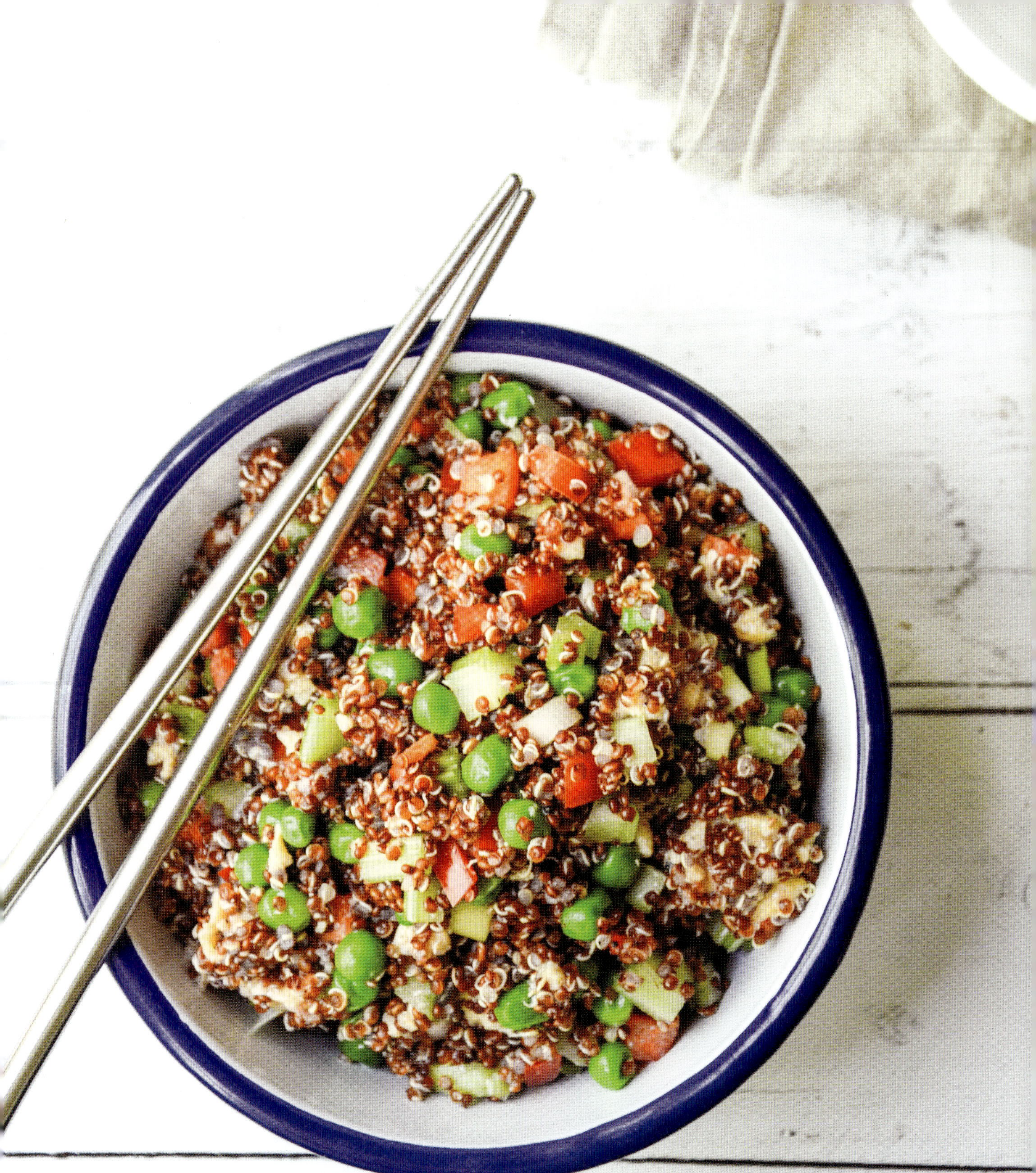

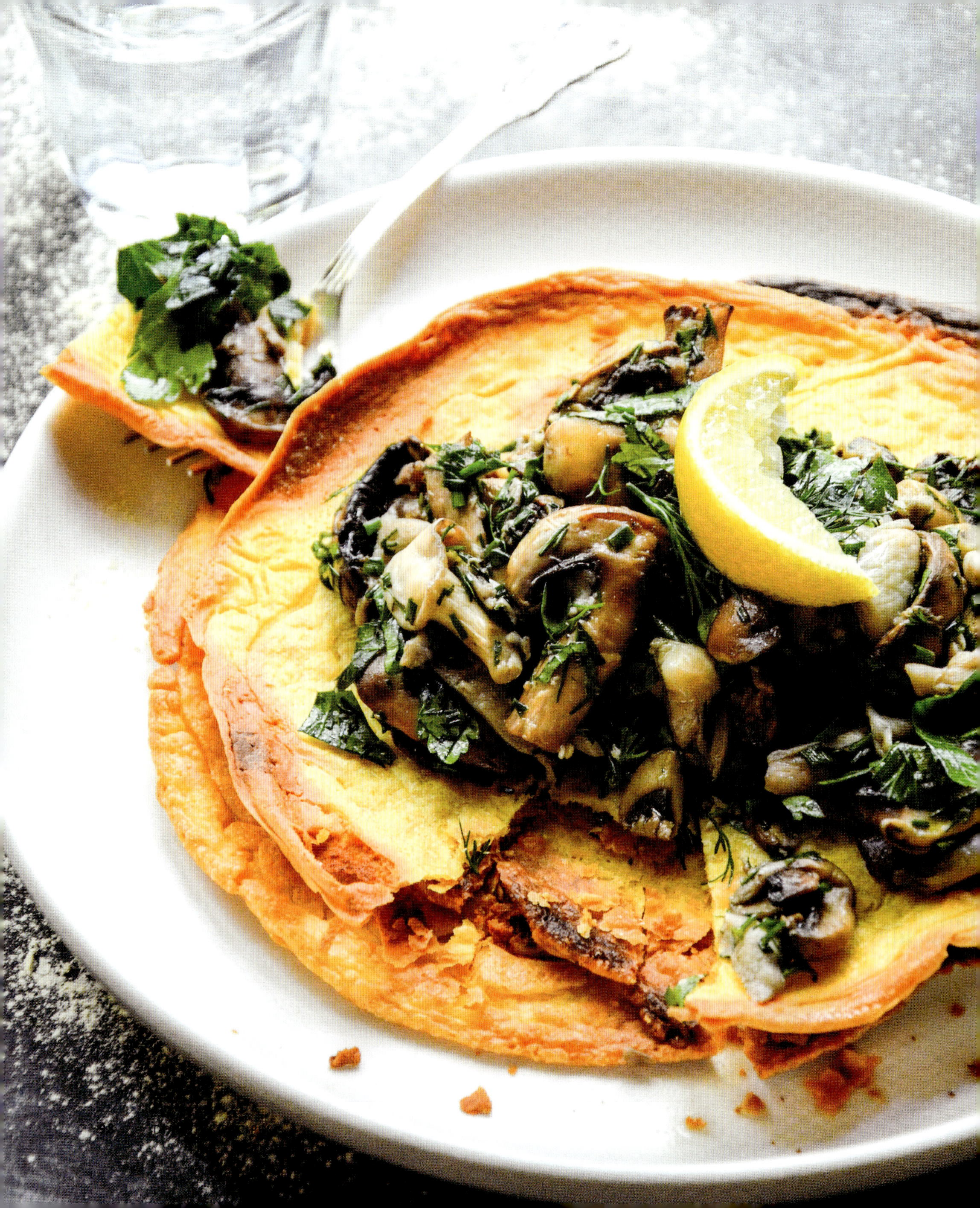

Herbed mushrooms on socca

Chickpea flour is a great staple to have on hand in the pantry for when you feel like a crispy, gluten free bread-pancake hybrid to top with delicious vegetables, or even to dip into a soup or curry sauce. Socca flatbread is simple to make and oh so delicious, add a combination of spices or herbs to the base recipe to adjust the flavour.

SERVES 4

SOCCA

1 cup (130g) chickpea flour/besan flour

1 cup (250ml) filtered water

1 tsp sea salt

2 tbsp extra virgin olive oil, plus more for the pan

HERBED MUSHROOMS

600g/1.3 lb mixed mushrooms, any variety

1 cup (40g) fresh flat leaf parsley, finely chopped

1 cup (50g) fresh dill, finely chopped

Juice from 1 lemon

Sea salt and black pepper

1 Prepare the socca by whisking the flour, water, salt and oil together in a bowl and letting it sit for 30 minutes.

2 Slice the mushrooms and add to a hot pan with 1 tbsp of extra virgin olive oil. Cook over medium heat until the mushrooms have softened and reduced in size. Take the pan off the heat and stir through the parsley, dill, lemon juice, a good pinch of sea salt and pepper. Taste and adjust seasoning if needed.

3 Heat the grill/broiler in your oven and place a cast iron pan or an oven safe dish/pan under the heat for 5 minutes. Carefully remove the pan using oven gloves, add a small amount of olive oil, just enough to coat the pan when you tilt it, then ladle in the batter and spread it around to form a thin layer. Place the pan back under the grill to cook for 5–7 minutes or until the bread turns golden brown. Remove from the oven and check the underside of the socca using a spatula, you may need to flip it over and cook the other side for a couple of minutes or it may be okay.

4 Serve the socca with the herbed mushrooms piled on top and additional fresh lemon juice if desired.

Sweet potato, black bean + jalapeño burger patties

Make these patties ahead of time and freeze individual portions for easy access. Add to a salad for lunch or go for the full burger, whether in a bun or lettuce leaves for a wheat free version. You can omit the jalapeño and replace with different spices, such as cumin or garam masala for a different taste.

MAKES 10

2 large sweet potatoes

1 cup (180g) cooked quinoa

1 cup (170g) cooked black beans

½ brown onion, diced

½ cup (20g) coriander/cilantro leaves, finely chopped

2 jalapñeo peppers, finely chopped

1 tbsp smoked paprika

1 tsp ground cumin

Pinch of salt and pepper

1 Preheat the oven to 180°C/350°F and line an oven tray with baking paper. Cut the sweet potatoes in half, drizzle with olive oil and a pinch of sea salt and roast for 40 minutes or until tender. Set aside to cool then scoop the soft flesh into a bowl and mash with a fork.

2 Thoroughly rinse the quinoa under water to remove any bitterness then add to a pan with 2 cups (500ml) of water and a pinch of salt over a medium heat. Cook until the quinoa has absorbed the water, about 15 minutes, then fluff with a fork and set aside to cool.

3 Add the cooked quinoa, black beans, onion, coriander, jalapeño peppers, smoked paprika, cumin and a good pinch of sea salt and black pepper to the bowl of sweet potato. Mix together until all ingredients and spices are evenly distributed.

4 Line an oven tray with fresh baking paper. Form the mixture into even-sized balls then place on the tray and push down to flatten each into a burger pattie shape. Bake for 30 minutes or until crisp, flipping the patties over halfway through.

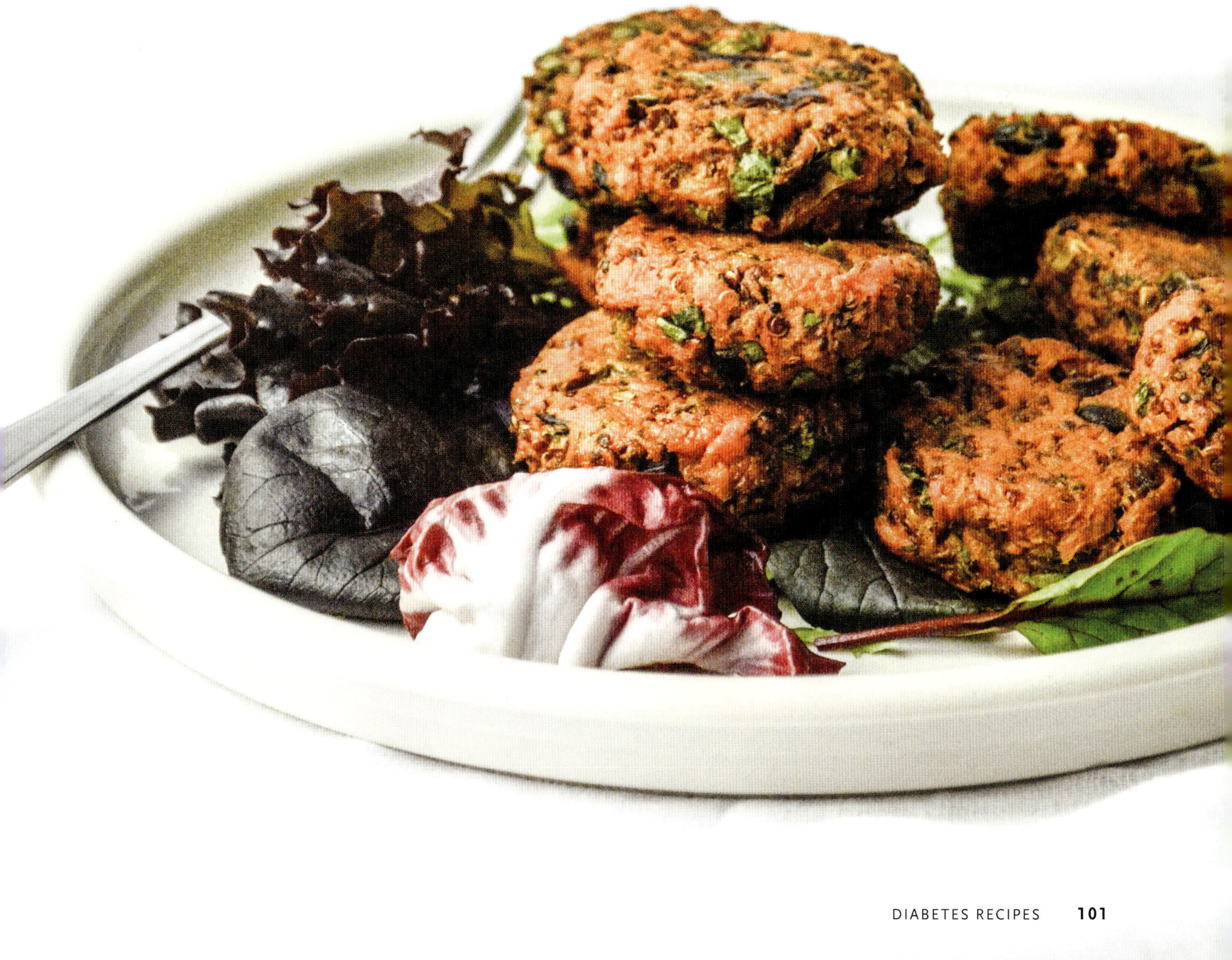

Pulled cider pork with roasted garlic + apple salad

This is a great dish to share with a group of people and really only needs a little preparation the night before cooking.

SERVES 6

PULLED PORK

1.5kg/3.3 lb boneless pork shoulder

½ cup (125ml) apple cider vinegar

1 cup (250ml) chicken stock

2 garlic cloves, minced

1 tbsp sea salt

¼ cup (60ml) raw honey

1 tsp mustard seeds

1½ tbsp smoked paprika

2 tsp sea salt

ROASTED GARLIC + APPLE SALAD

1 garlic bulb

2 green apples

¼ cup (60ml) lemon juice

250g/9 oz salad greens, such as baby spinach, rocket/arugula, watercress

2 tbsp extra virgin olive oil

1 Place the pork in a large plastic ziplock bag or in a large bowl.

2 In a bowl, combine the apple cider vinegar, chicken stock, garlic, salt and honey, whisk until combined.

3 In a small, dry pan toast the mustard seeds for 2 minutes until they begin to pop. Add the mustard seeds to the cider vinegar mixture and stir through. Pour the marinade over the pork shoulder. If using a bag, seal the bag and massage the marinade around the meat. If using a bowl, turn the pork over a couple of times in the liquid before resting it flesh (not skin) side down and covering the bowl with plastic wrap. Place in the fridge overnight.

4 Remove the pork from the fridge at least half an hour before cooking. Mix the smoked paprika and sea salt together then rub over the flesh side of the pork (not the skin).

5 To cook the pork you can use a pressure cooker (cooking time 2–2.5 hours on high) with some of the marinade liquid at the bottom of the bowl, a cast iron pot in the oven (heat the oven to 160°C/320°F and cook low and slow, for approximately 4 hours with a little of the liquid in the bottom of the pan), or on a BBQ (4–5 hours).

6 To test if the pork is ready, use two forks to shred some of the meat, if it comes off easily the muscle meat has broken down enough and you can set the meat aside to shred, discard the skin. If it is still tough, cook for a further 30 minutes and check again.

7 Prepare the salad by preheating the oven to 180°C/350°F and lining an oven tray with baking paper. Cut the top off the garlic bulb and place the bulb on the tray, drizzle with a little olive oil and roast for 20–30 minutes until the cloves are soft and beginning to caramelise. Remove from the oven and set aside to cool.

8 Core the apples and finely slice, either into crescents or matchsticks. Lightly coat the apple in lemon juice to stop it from browning.

9 In a bowl combine the salad leaves, roasted garlic and apple slices then drizzle the extra virgin olive oil over the top and serve alongside the pulled pork.

Chicken + avocado skewers

Adding avocado to these skewers not only boosts the healthy fats content of the recipe but also delivers a rich, creamy textual variation.

MAKES 6

350g/12 oz chicken breast fillets

1 Spanish/red onion (optional)

¼ cup (60ml) extra virgin olive oil

1 tbsp dried oregano

1 tsp sea salt

1-2 avocados, depending on size

6 wooden skewers

1 lemon

1 Preheat a BBQ hotplate or grill while you prepare the skewers. It's best to soak the wooden skewers overnight in water to prevent them from burning while cooking. If you can't do this, soak them for as long as possible before threading the chicken on.

2 Slice the chicken into long thin strips or into cubes. If using, peel the onion and chop into chunky wedges. Add the chicken and onion to a bowl with the extra virgin olive oil, oregano and sea salt. Use a spoon or tongs to toss the mixture so the chicken is evenly coated.

3 Slice the avocado in half and remove the pit and skin. Dice the avocado flesh into cubes and set aside.

4 Take each skewer and thread on a piece of chicken followed by an onion wedge and some avocado. Top the skewer with another piece of chicken and place on a plate. Once the BBQ or grill is hot, cook the skewers for 10 minutes or until cooked through. Thinner strips of chicken will cook faster, for chicken cubes cook for an additional few minutes before checking to see if it's cooked through.

5 Cut the lemon in half and drizzle fresh lemon juice over the top of the skewers before serving.

Sweet potato noodle stir-fry

Spiralising sweet potato will give you a sturdy noodle ideal for using in stir-fries and a healthier alternative to wheat noodles. Prep all of your ingredients before you begin cooking, heat the wok up and you'll have a meal ready in minutes, it really is a quicker and healthier option to fast food.

SERVES 1

1 medium sweet potato

3 large mushrooms, any variety

1½ cups (100g) kale or other leafy greens

1 spring onion/scallion

1 free range egg

1 tbsp Tamari/wheat free soy sauce

1 tsp black pepper

1 Peel the sweet potato, spiralise into noodles and set aside.

2 Roughly chop the mushrooms, kale and spring onion and set aside.

3 Crack the egg and lightly whisk it.

4 Heat up a wok with 1 tbsp of coconut oil. Add the egg, mushrooms, kale and spring onion and cook for 30 seconds, stirring with a wooden spoon or spatula. Add the sweet potato noodles, the Tamari and black pepper. Cook for 4–5 minutes, adding a dash of water if needed to keep the mixture loose from the wok.

You can pre-steam the sweet potato noodles before adding them to the wok if you would prefer a tenderer noodle, while adding it straight to the wok will help the noodles retain their shape and texture.

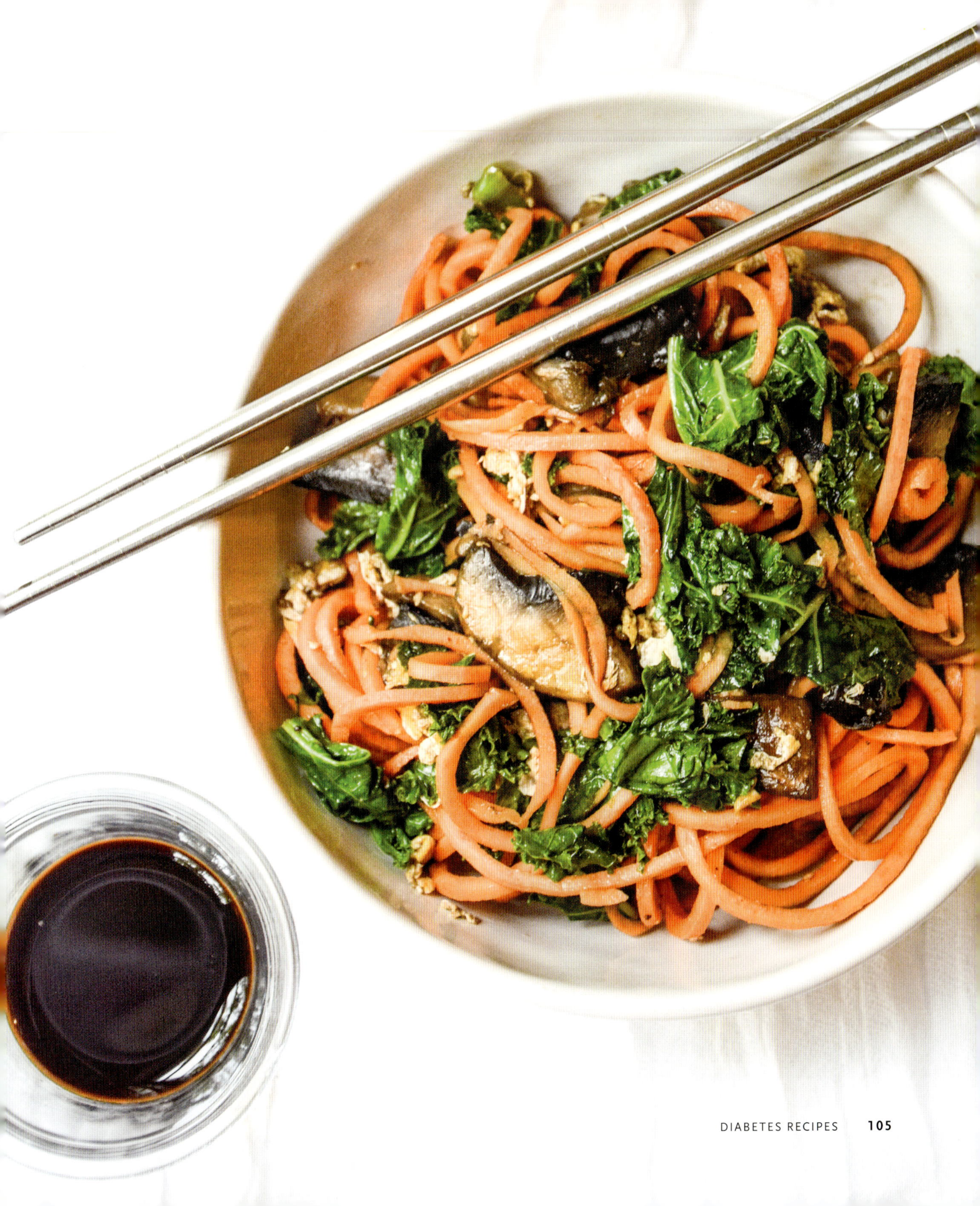

Roast paprika chicken

A roast chicken is a real crowd pleaser, perfect for a Sunday lunch with the family or an intimate dinner for two, after which leftovers turn into delicious lunches. Store bought roast chickens can be handy for busy days or hot weather when you don't want to use your oven, but unless you know how they cook their chickens you may find a host of unnecessary ingredients added. From the stuffing to the seasoning on the skin, you can count on a store bought chicken being higher in sodium than one you cook at home. Aim to only buy free range chicken, it's more expensive but the quality of the meat is sensational.

SERVES 4–6

1 large chicken (weight will vary, approximately 1.2–1.5kg/2.6–3.3lb)

1 lemon

1 small bunch of thyme

Sea salt and black pepper

2 tbsp smoked paprika (or regular paprika)

Extra virgin olive oil

1 Prep the chicken by removing it from the refrigerator one hour before cooking and allowing it to come to room temperature. Use a paper towel to pat the skin dry.

2 Preheat the oven to 180°C/350°F.

3 Slice the lemon in half and fill the chicken's cavity with the lemon and thyme. It can be easier to do this while holding the chicken upside down. Sprinkle in some sea salt and black pepper. Tie the legs together (if not done already) with some butcher's string.

4 Place the chicken in a roasting pan. You can elevate the chicken on a shelf within the pan or if you don't have one place some additional thyme sprigs in the bottom of the pan before laying the chicken over the top.

5 Sprinkle the paprika over the top of the chicken, including the wings and legs. Follow this with a moderate sprinkling (approximately 1 tbsp) of sea salt and a good grinding of fresh black pepper. Drizzle extra virgin olive oil over the chicken and massage the seasoning into the skin.

6 Place the chicken in the oven and, depending on weight, cook for approximately 1½ hours, testing the chicken is cooked by using a meat thermometer, cutting into the chicken, or piercing the chicken and seeing if the juices run clear. As always with chicken, if in doubt cook for a little bit longer to avoid undercooked meat.

7 Make sure to baste the chicken every twenty minutes during cooking to avoid dry or burnt skin.

8 Serve roast chicken with a side salad such as leafy greens, julienned cucumber and dutch carrots, or roasted seasonal vegetables.

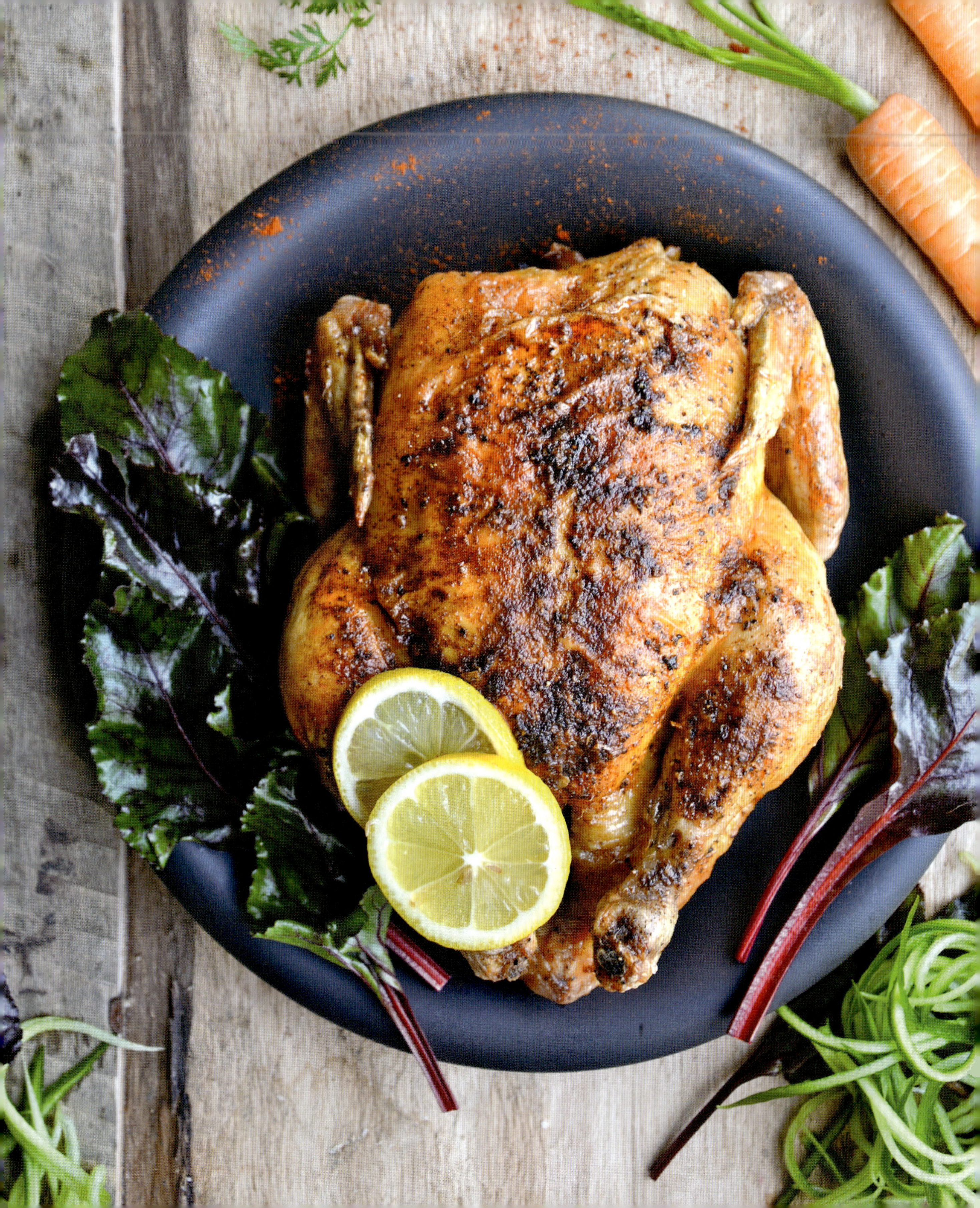

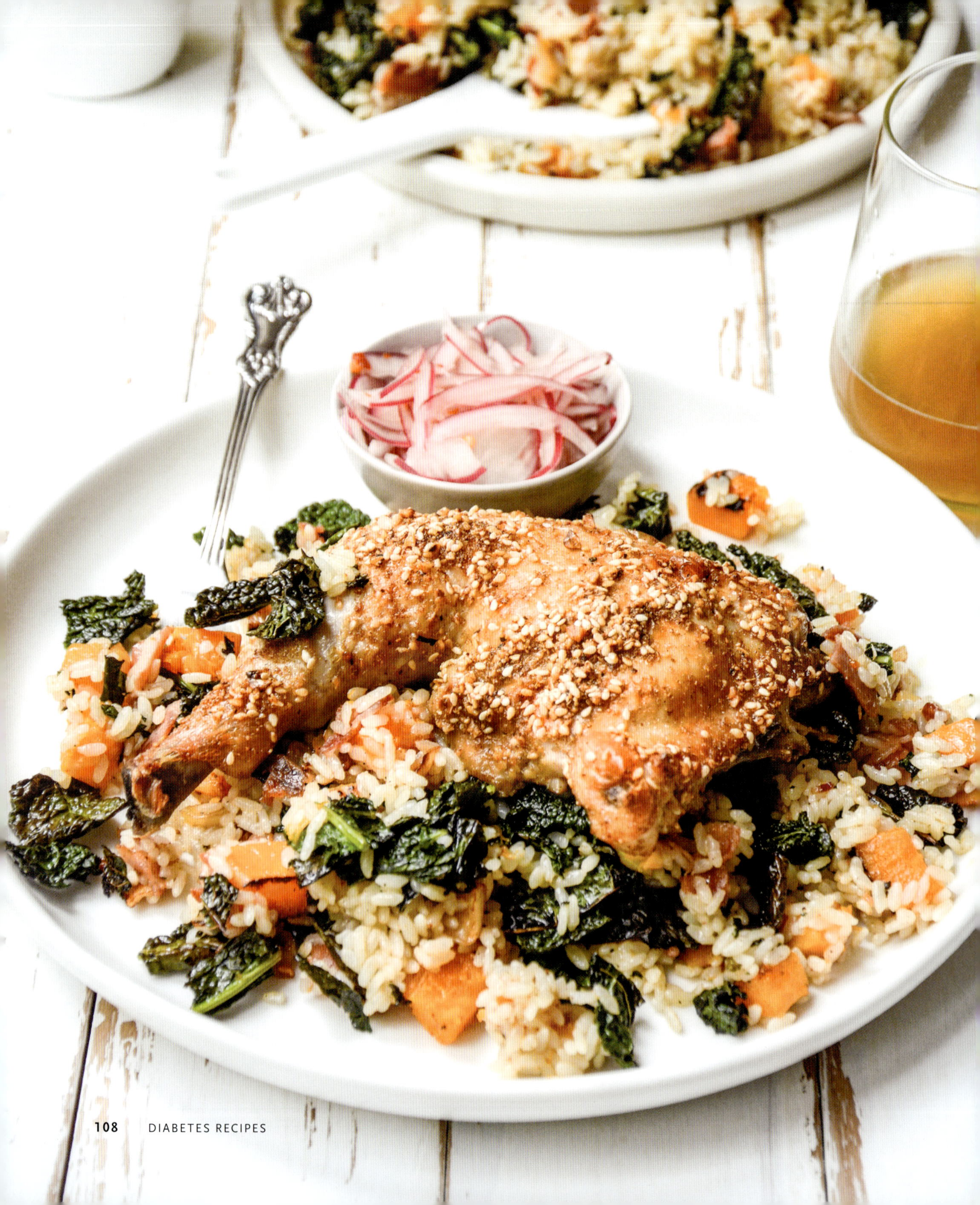

Dukkah crusted chicken maryland with confetti rice

SERVES 4

3 chicken marylands (the thigh and drumstick portion)

2 cups (500ml) chicken stock

Handful of fresh thyme sprigs

DUKKAH

½ cup (40g) sesame seeds

2 tbsp coriander seeds

2 tbsp cumin seeds

1 tsp sea salt

Pinch of black peppercorns

CONFETTI RICE

1 cup (200g) medium grain rice

1½–2 cups (375–500ml) chicken stock

6 slices of pancetta

½ medium bunch of Tuscan kale

400g/14 oz pumpkin, any variety

2 tsp smoked paprika

1 tsp sea salt

Freshly ground black pepper

QUICK PICKLED ONION

1 large Spanish/red onion

¼ cup (60ml) apple cider vinegar

2 tbsp rice wine vinegar

1 One hour before cooking, place the chicken, stock and thyme in a bowl or tray. Turn the chicken several times to coat. Cover the bowl with cling film and place in the refrigerator.

2 Preheat the oven to 180°C/350°F.

3 Drizzle a small amount of olive oil into a pan over medium heat and cook the marylands for 5 minutes before turning them and cooking for a further 5 minutes. Transfer the chicken to an ovenproof dish and roast in the oven for 20 minutes or until cooked through.

4 While the chicken is cooking prepare the rice. Using a rice cooker or the absorption method on the stovetop, cook the rice with the chicken stock until fluffy. Roughly dice the pancetta and cook in a small pan with a drizzle of olive oil. Once crisp, set aside on a plate lined with paper towel.

5 Dice the pumpkin into even cubes and steam for 5 minutes then toss through the smoked paprika and sea salt. Add a drizzle of olive oil to the same pan you cooked the pancetta in and add the pumpkin. Cook for a further 5 minutes until slightly caramelised.

6 Remove the Tuscan kale leaves from the stem (discarding the stem) and cut into rough chunks. Place the kale in a bowl and drizzle over a small amount of olive oil. Use your hands to massage the oil into the leaves for a minute until the leaves start to soften. Place the leaves on an oven tray lined with baking paper and roast in the oven alongside the chicken for 10 minutes or until crisp, checking it every few minutes to make sure it doesn't burn.

7 Prepare the quick pickled onion by peeling the onion, cutting it in half and finely slicing it into half crescents. Using a mandolin slicer makes this easy and uniform but you can also use a knife. Place the onion in a bowl and add the apple cider and rice wine vinegars. Toss the onion to coat in the liquid and let sit until ready to serve. Toss the onions every 5 minutes to help them absorb the liquid and soften. You can make the pickled onion ahead of time for extra soft onions but they should be soft after soaking for about 15 minutes.

8 When the rice is cooked spoon it into a large serving dish and stir through the crispy pancetta, roasted pumpkin and crispy kale; taste and season with black pepper or additional salt if needed. Serve the chicken atop the confetti rice with the quick pickled onion on the side.

Cashew satay beef skewers

These beef skewers use top quality meat, although you can substitute with whatever you have access to. Using a quality eye fillet cut will ensure these are tender and melt in the mouth.

MAKES 12 SMALL

400–500g/14–18oz eye fillet beef

2 tbsp mustard of choice (optional)

2 tbsp extra virgin olive oil

2 garlic cloves, minced

Pinch of sea salt

SATAY SAUCE

1 cup (125g) cashews, soaked in water overnight

¼ cup (60ml) fresh lemon juice

1 tbsp tamari/wheat free soy sauce

½ cup (125ml) hulled tahini

2 garlic cloves

Sea salt and black pepper

1 Preheat a barbecue or a grill plate while you prepare the kebabs.

2 Remove any visible fat from the edge of the beef. Cube the eye fillet into an even number of chunks.

3 Use 12 small wooden skewers(soak overnight in water to prevent burning) and thread the beef evenly onto each. Keep the meat pushed close together. You can add additional ingredients to the kebab if you choose, such as slices of onion or red capsicum.

4 Prepare the marinade by whisking together the mustard (if using), extra virgin olive oil, minced garlic, sea salt and black pepper. Brush each kebab with the marinade until all used up.

5 By now the barbecue or grill plate should be hot. Cook the kebabs for 3-4 minutes each side then remove and set aside to rest for 5 minutes.

6 Prepare the satay sauce by rinsing the soaked cashews in fresh water, straining in a sieve then adding to the bowl of a food processor along with the lemon juice, tamari, tahini, garlic, and a pinch of salt and pepper. Blitz until a smooth paste forms, adding a touch of water as needed to thin the consistency. For a nut-free satay sauce, omit the cashews and increase the tahini to 1 cup (250ml).

7 Serve with a side salad and the satay sauce drizzled over the top of the kebabs or in a small container for dipping.

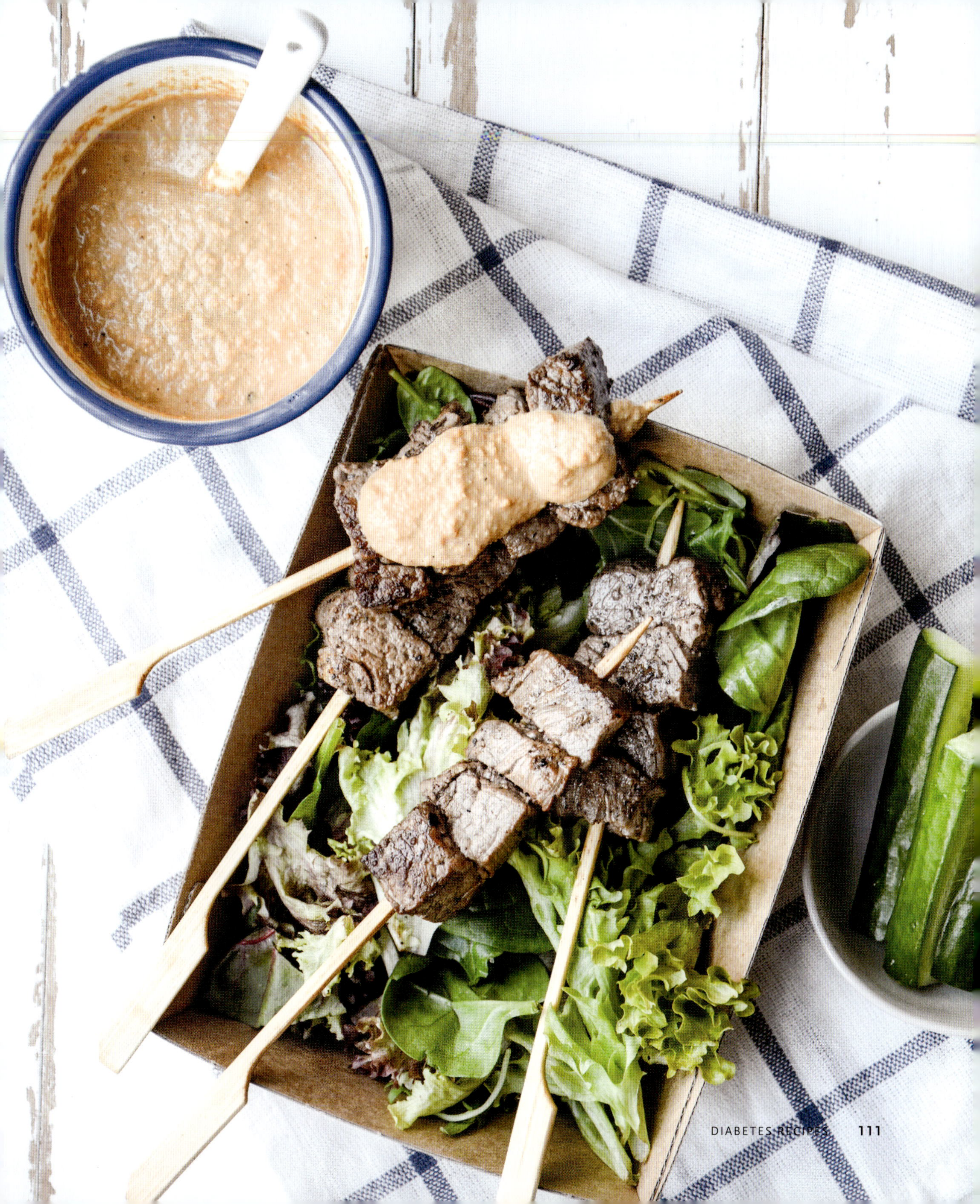

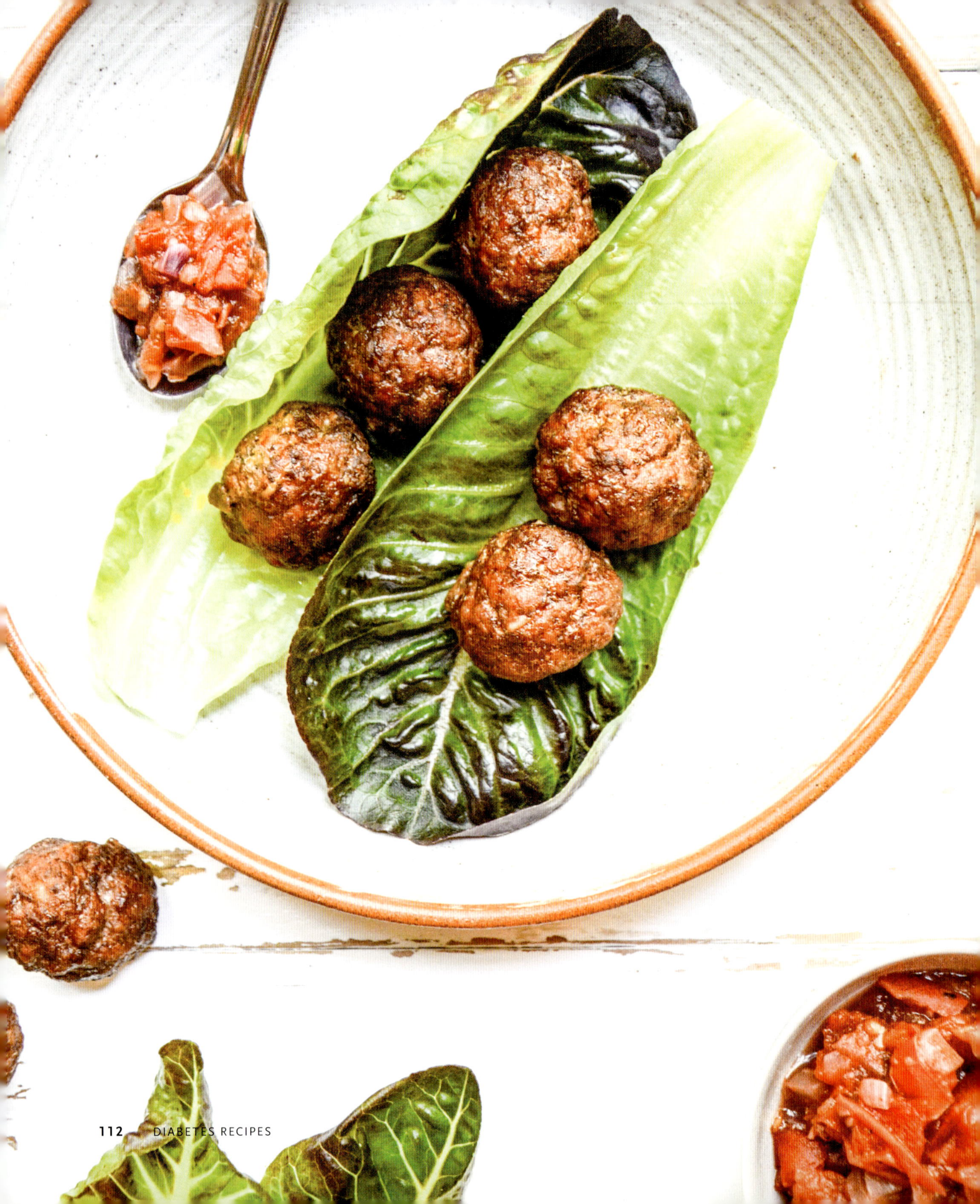

Meatball subs with tomato relish

Meatballs are an easy meal or snack and you can keep the seasoning simple or add spices or herbs to make the flavour more interesting. Serving the meatballs in crisp lettuce cups is perfect for lunch on the go, picnics, parties or just as a bread-free sandwich option. You can make the meatballs and relish ahead of time and freeze for busy days.

SERVES 4-6

500g/1 lb minced beef

½ Spanish/red onion, finely diced

1 tbsp smoked paprika

1 iceberg or cos lettuce, leaves removed

TOMATO RELISH

4 tomatoes, diced

2 garlic cloves, minced

2 tbsp white wine vinegar

1 tbsp apple cider vinegar

½ tsp all spice

Pinch of salt and pepper

1 Preheat the oven to 180°C/350°F.

2 In a bowl combine the minced beef, onion and smoked paprika. Roll the mixture into small balls and place on an oven tray lined with baking paper. Bake in the oven for 15-20 minutes until cooked through.

3 Prepare the tomato relish by adding all the ingredients to a pan over medium heat. Cook for 20–30 minutes until the tomatoes are soft and the mixture has thickened.

4 Serve the meatballs in lettuce leaves with a spoonful of relish on top.

These meatballs go great with zucchini noodles, steamed or roasted vegetables, or on top of a fresh salad.

Instant noodle pots

Quick noodles with flavour sachets are a popular meal option for many as they're cheap and flavourful. They're also usually jam-packed with high levels of salt and artificial ingredients. Making instant noodle pots at home is incredibly easy and much healthier than the store-bought variety.

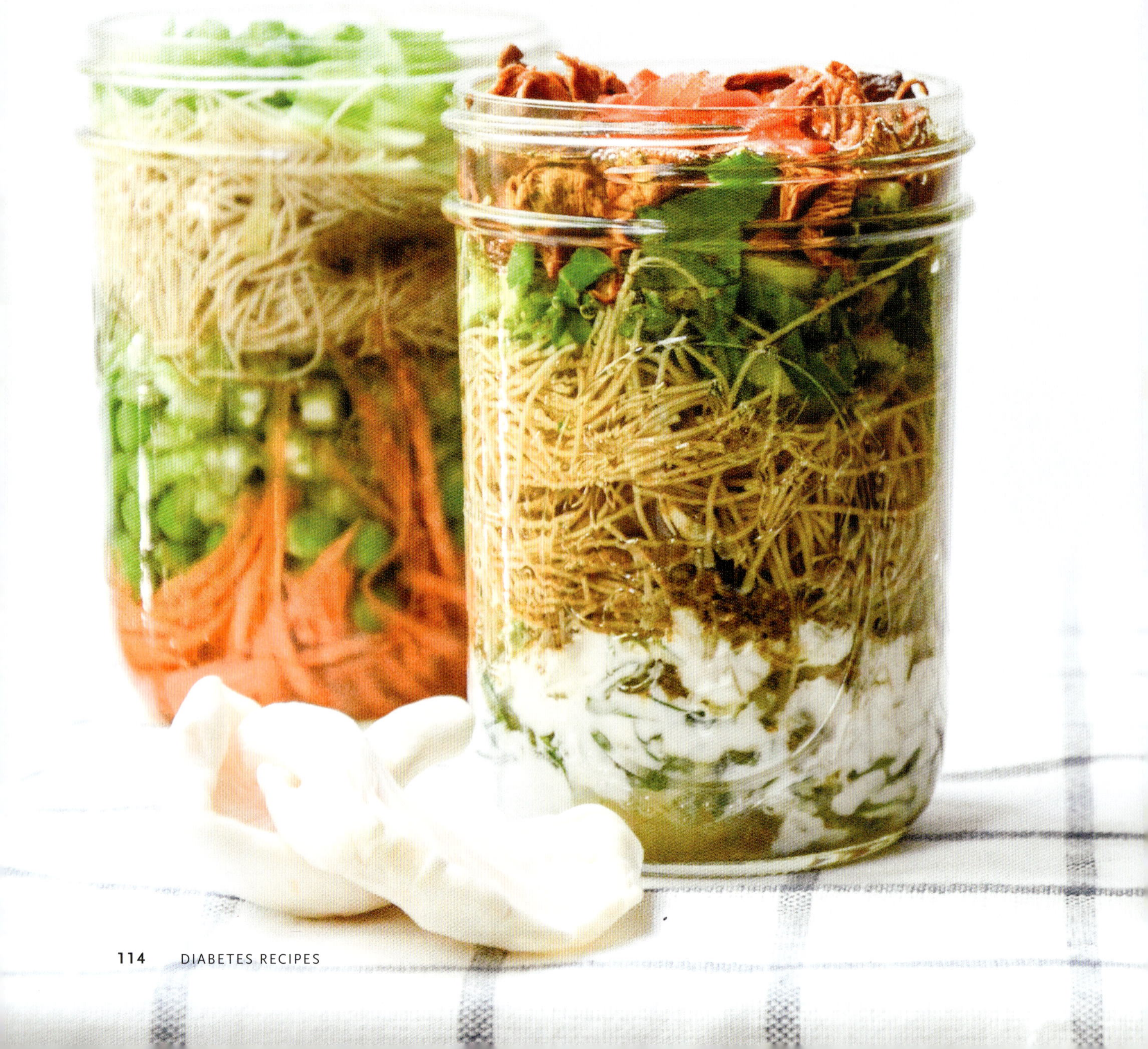

Spring vegetable

SERVES 1

½ carrot, grated

½ cup (65g) frozen peas

1 celery stick, diced

1 spring onion/scallion, diced

1 tsp ground cumin

½ tsp curry powder

1 tsp sea salt

50g/1.8 oz brown rice or white vermicelli noodles

1 cup (250ml) boiling water

Add the carrot, peas, celery, spring onion, cumin, curry powder and sea salt to a jar. Place the lid on and shake to combine the flavours. Remove the lid, add the noodles and reseal the jar. When ready to eat, pour in the boiling water until the contents are just covered. Let the jar sit for 2 minutes for the noodles to soften and the vegetables to heat through.

Creamy mushroom

SERVES 1

⅓ cup (80ml) coconut milk

1 bok choy bulb

Handful of oyster mushrooms

Handful of dried porcini mushrooms (optional)

1 tsp garam masala

1 tsp sea salt

50g/1.8 oz brown or white vermicelli noodles

1 cup (250ml) boiling water

Pour the coconut milk into the bottom of a jar. Finely slice the bok choy and oyster mushrooms and add to the jar followed by the dried porcini mushrooms if using. Dust over the garam masala and sea salt then add the noodles. Pour in the boiling water, wait 2 minutes then stir the contents of the jar so everything is evenly distributed.

Pan seared salmon with dill pea mash

Cooking fresh salmon at home is incredibly easy and always delivers tasty results. You don't need to be fancy with flavours or sides, the classic pairing of lemon and dill in this recipe helps the natural flavour of the salmon shine.

SERVES 2

2 medium salmon fillets

1 tsp sea salt

1 tsp black pepper

Zest of 1 lemon

Extra virgin olive oil

3 cups (385g) peas

250g/9oz broccolini

1 tbsp unsalted butter

¼ cup (25g) fresh dill, finely chopped

1 Season each salmon fillet with sea salt, black pepper and lemon zest. Drizzle with extra virgin olive oil and set aside.

2 Heat a frying pan over a medium heat and add the salmon skin side down. Cook for 4 minutes each side.

3 While the salmon is cooking, steam the peas and broccolini until tender then stir through the butter and dill. Set the broccolini aside and mash the peas roughly with a fork or using a food processor to create a creamier mash.

4 Serve the salmon fillets on top of the pea mash and alongside the broccolini. Squeeze fresh lemon juice over the top.

Other great sources of Omega 3s include walnuts, flaxseeds, pumpkin seeds, Brussels sprouts, cauliflower, eggs, grass-fed beef, kale, spinach and parsley.

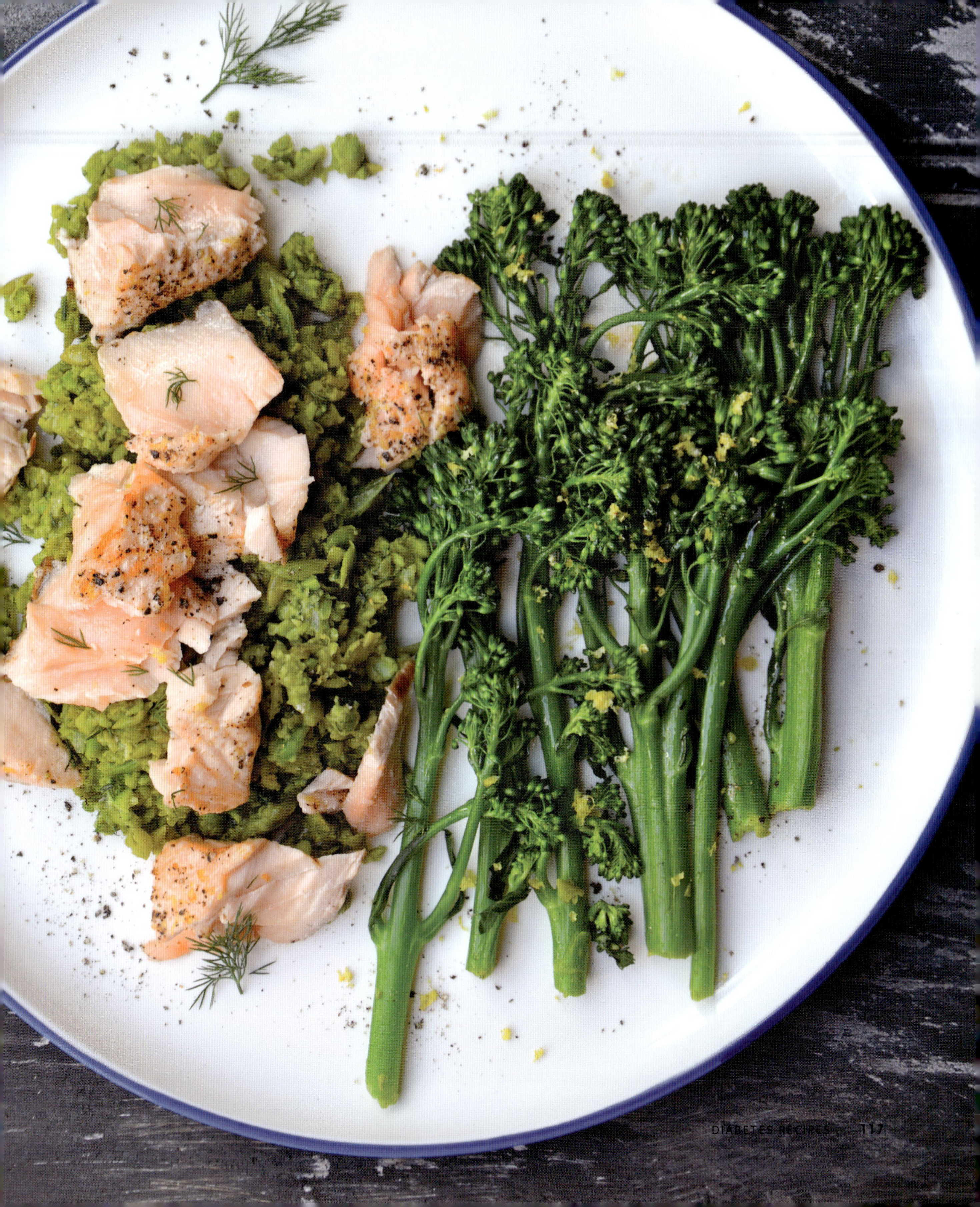

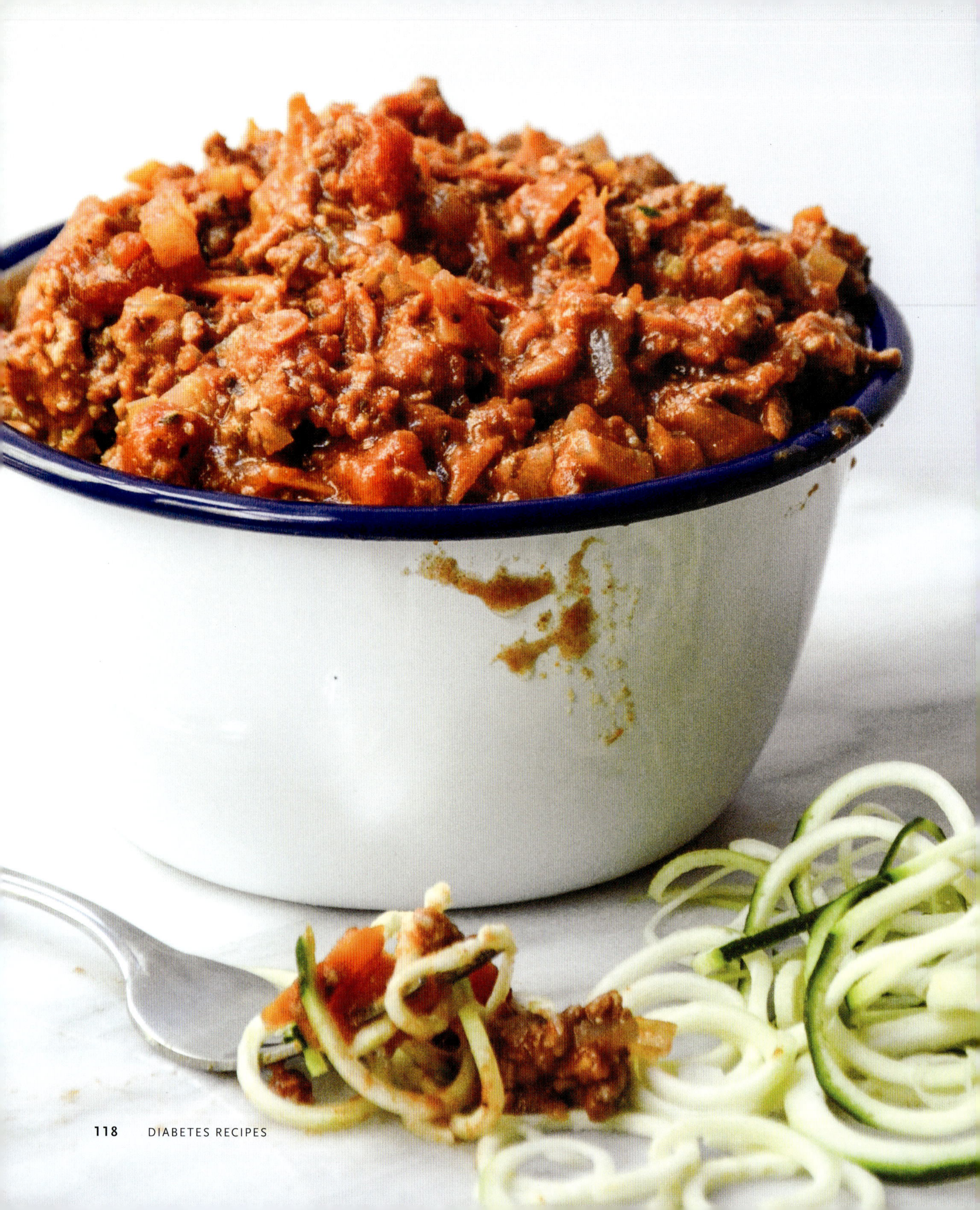

Veg packed bolognaise

This recipe is a great opportunity to pack in extra vegetables with a sweet tomato sauce. Whether you serve this traditionally with wheat noodles or opt for rice noodles, spiralised vegetable noodles, or simply serve the meat sauce over the top of steamed vegetables, you'll find it's a real crowd pleaser.

SERVES 4

1 brown onion
4 garlic cloves
400g/14 oz minced beef
1 large carrot
200g/7 oz pumpkin, any variety
1 zucchini/courgette
2 celery stalks
1 can of crushed tomatoes
1 tbsp dried basil
2 tbsp red wine or red wine vinegar
Sea salt and black pepper

1. Finely dice the brown onion, crush the garlic and add to a large pan with a drizzle of extra virgin olive oil. Cook over a medium heat until the onion softens then add the minced beef and cook until browned.
2. Grate the carrot, pumpkin and zucchini and add to the pot. Finely dice the celery and add to the pot, stir so that all the vegetables are mixed with the meat.
3. Add the tomatoes then fill the can with water and add to the pot.
4. Add the dried basil, red wine and a good pinch of sea salt and ground black pepper. Stir to combine then reduce the heat to low and let the sauce simmer for 45 minutes.
5. Serve with spiralised zucchini noodles or pasta of choice.

drinks

Cucumber chia smoothie
Coconut + cucumber lemonade
Choc malt cacao nib crunch
Golden turmeric milk
Turmeric + carrot juice
Super greens juice
Lemon, lime + ACV
Ginger + lemon thyme fizz
Basic nut milk
Oat milk
Coconut milk
Pina colada
Almond, Brazil and cashew butter

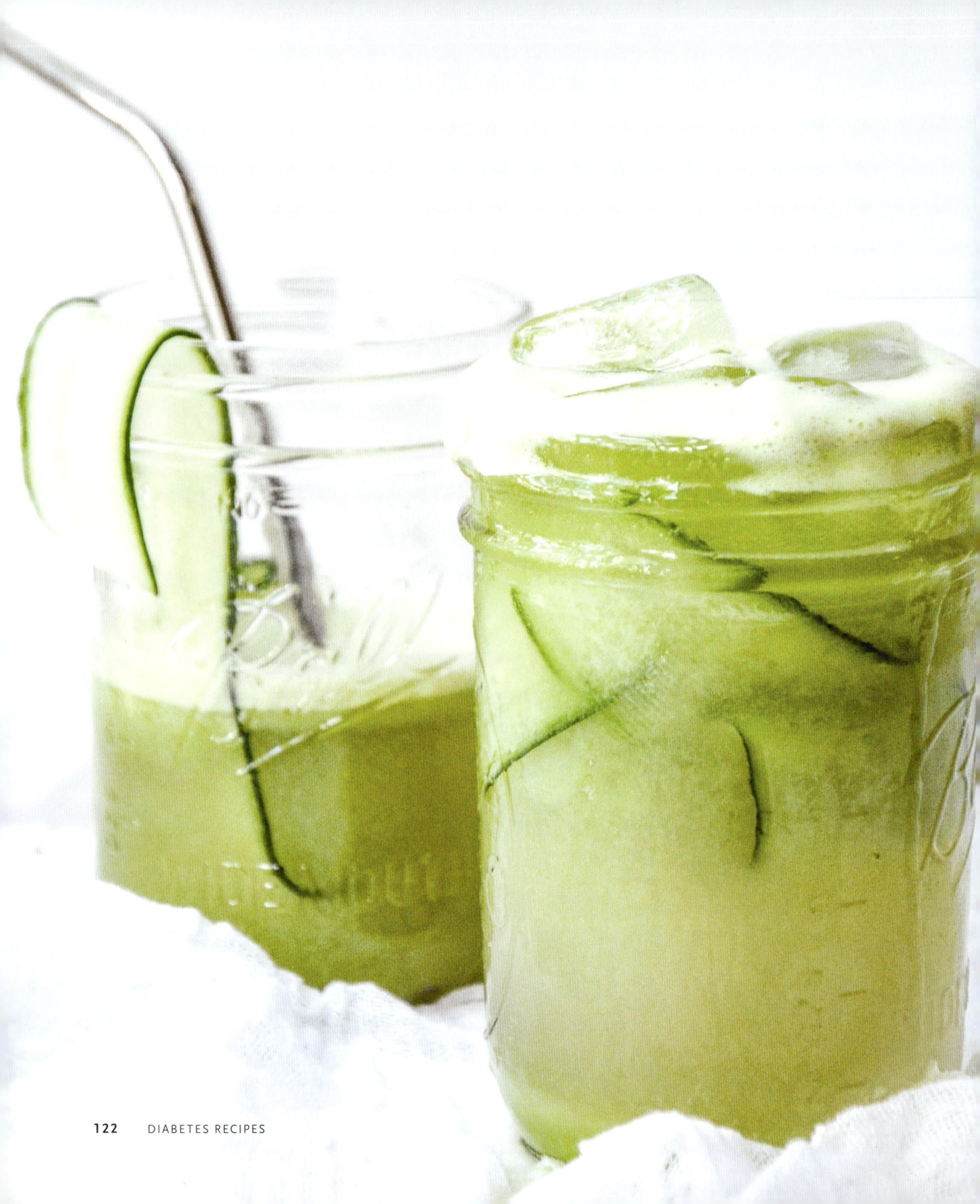

Cucumber chia smoothie

Cucumber is a fantastic hydrating ingredient to add to smoothies and juices. Combine cucumber in this smoothie with an apple for sweetness and chia seeds for fibre and protein, and you have a delicious and energising drink to kick start your day or boost your energy in the afternoon.

SERVES 2

1 tbsp chia seeds

½ cup (125ml) filtered water

1 cucumber, any variety, diced

1 cup (30g) green leaves of choice

½ an apple

1 tbsp nut butter (optional)

2 cups (500ml) milk of choice

Soak the chia seeds in the water for 15 minutes then add to a blender with the cucumber, green leaves, apple, nut butter and milk, blend on high until smooth.

Coconut + cucumber lemonade

This refreshing drink can be made as a juice or blended into a smoothie, depending on your preference. Add a small knob of fresh ginger root for an added bite and serve with plenty of ice and fresh mint sprigs.

SERVES 2

1 large cucumber

1 cup (160g) pineapple chunks, freeze the fruit if making a smoothie

Juice from 1 lemon

2 cups (500ml) coconut water

1 Juice the cucumber and pineapple in your juicer then add the lemon juice and coconut water to the jug and stir to thoroughly combine.

2 If making a smoothie, dice the cucumber into similar-sized chunks and add to the blender with the pineapple, lemon juice and coconut water. Blitz until smooth. You can replace the coconut water with coconut milk for an even creamier treat.

Choc malt cacao nib crunch

This healthy spin on the classic chocolate milkshake is a treasure trove of flavour thanks to a combination of raw cacao powder, vanilla powder and maca root powder. While maca can be omitted from the recipe if you choose, this ground root is rich in B vitamins as well as vitamins C and E. It's also a great hormone balancing ingredient rich in iron, zinc and magnesium.

SERVES 1

1½ cups (375ml) coconut milk

1½ tbsp maca root powder

1 tbsp raw cacao powder

½ tsp vanilla powder

1 tbsp cacao nibs, to serve (optional)

Add the coconut milk, maca root, raw cacao and vanilla powders to a blender and blitz on high until combined. Pour into a glass and serve with cacao nibs sprinkled on top.

Raw cacao is the unrefined version of the more common cocoa powder you see on supermarket shelves. Take the time to seek out raw cacao powder for your smoothies to maximise the nutritional benefits of this tasty food.

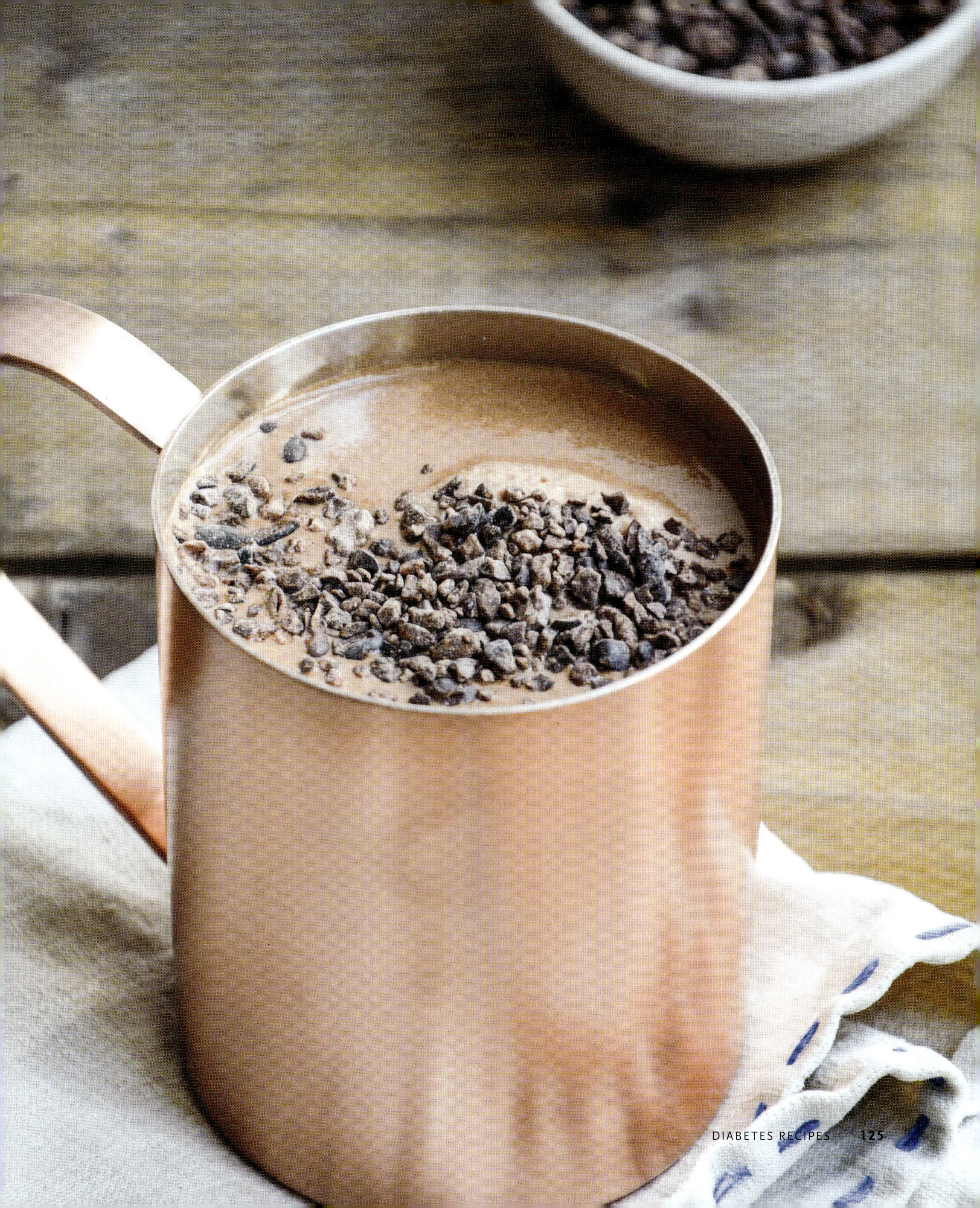

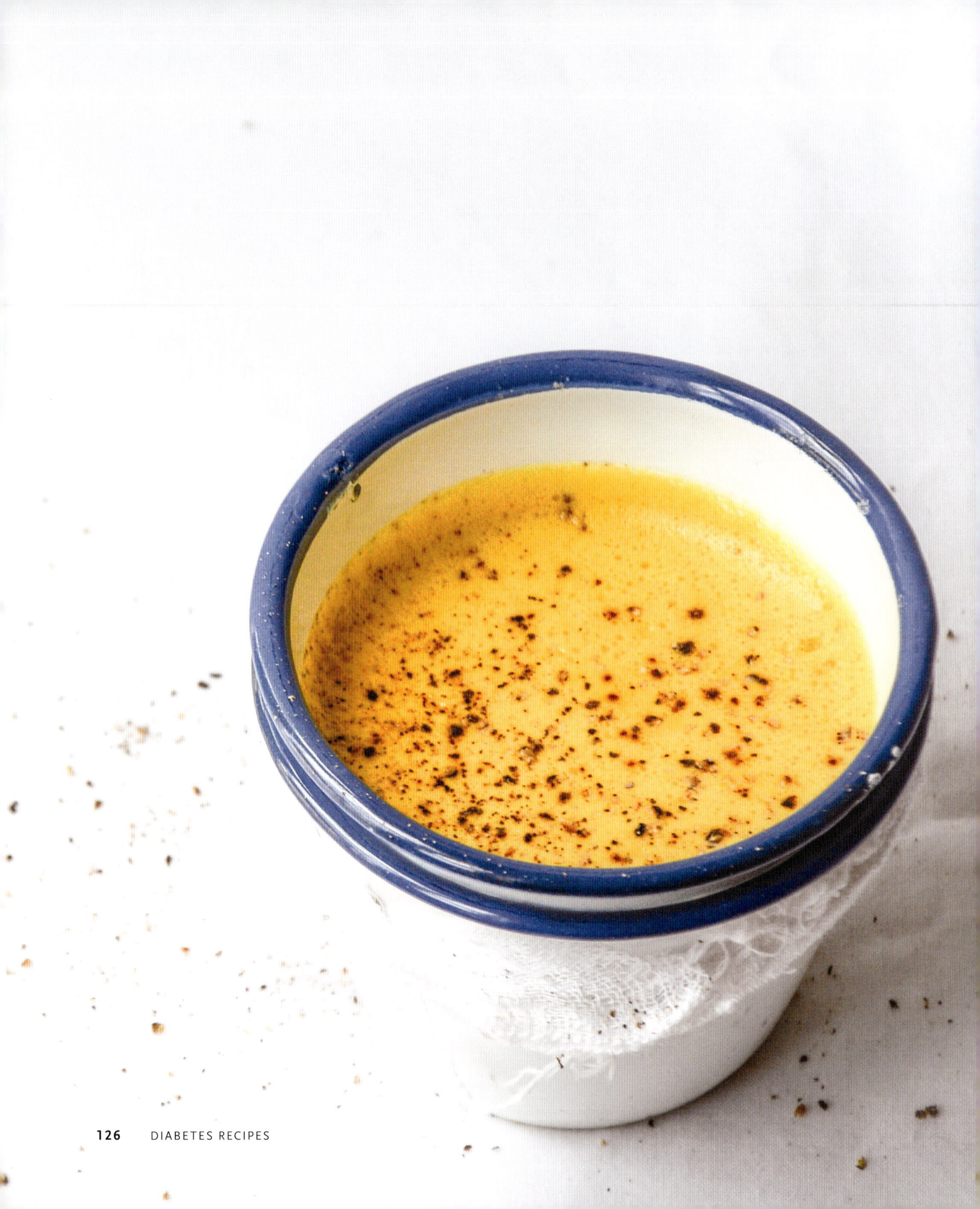

Golden turmeric milk

This warm drink is not only super nutritious but nourishing too. Turmeric is often known as a healing spice and is a strong antioxidant and anti-inflammatory high in manganese and iron that can be used to help treat everything from the common cold to an upset stomach. It is the curcumin found in turmeric that makes it such a powerful spice; adding pepper to the turmeric will help make the curcumin more readily available to your body.

SERVES 1

1 cup (250ml) milk of choice (almond, coconut etc)

1 tsp fresh or ground turmeric

½ tsp ground cinnamon

Pinch of freshly ground black pepper

Optional extras: 1 tbsp coconut oil, 1 tsp grated fresh ginger root, sweetener of choice (honey, maple syrup etc)

1 Add the milk, turmeric, cinnamon and black pepper to a small saucepan. If using the coconut oil, ginger or sweetener you can also add these now.

2 Whisk or use a handheld immersion blender to blitz the mixture together until smooth and golden in colour. Simmer over a low heat for 10 minutes. Serve warm.

If you find it hard to adjust to the taste of golden turmeric milk, add a small amount of a sweetener such as raw honey or maple syrup. Aim to reduce the amount of sweetener added each time until you can enjoy the drink sweetener free.

Turmeric + carrot juice

The power of turmeric in our diets cannot be underestimated; it really is a powerhouse spice that we should be aiming to include more of on a weekly if not daily basis. Unfortunately many of us are intimidated to use turmeric for fear of staining everything in sight a lovely shade of yellow. Turmeric's power as an anti-inflammatory is thanks to the active ingredient curcumin. Simply add a pinch of black pepper to help make the curcumin more bio-available to your body.

SERVES 1

1 large carrot
1 inch piece of fresh turmeric
1 inch piece of fresh ginger
4 celery stalks, leaves included
Pinch of ground black pepper

Feed the carrot and turmeric through the juicer first followed by the fresh ginger and celery stalks and leaves. Pour the juice into a glass and stir through the black pepper. Enjoy immediately.

If a turmeric spill occurs remain calm! Simply dilute equal parts water and bicarb soda in a small bowl then place a spoonful on the stain. Leave for 2 minutes then clean with a damp cloth. If the spill occurs on clothing wash immediately.

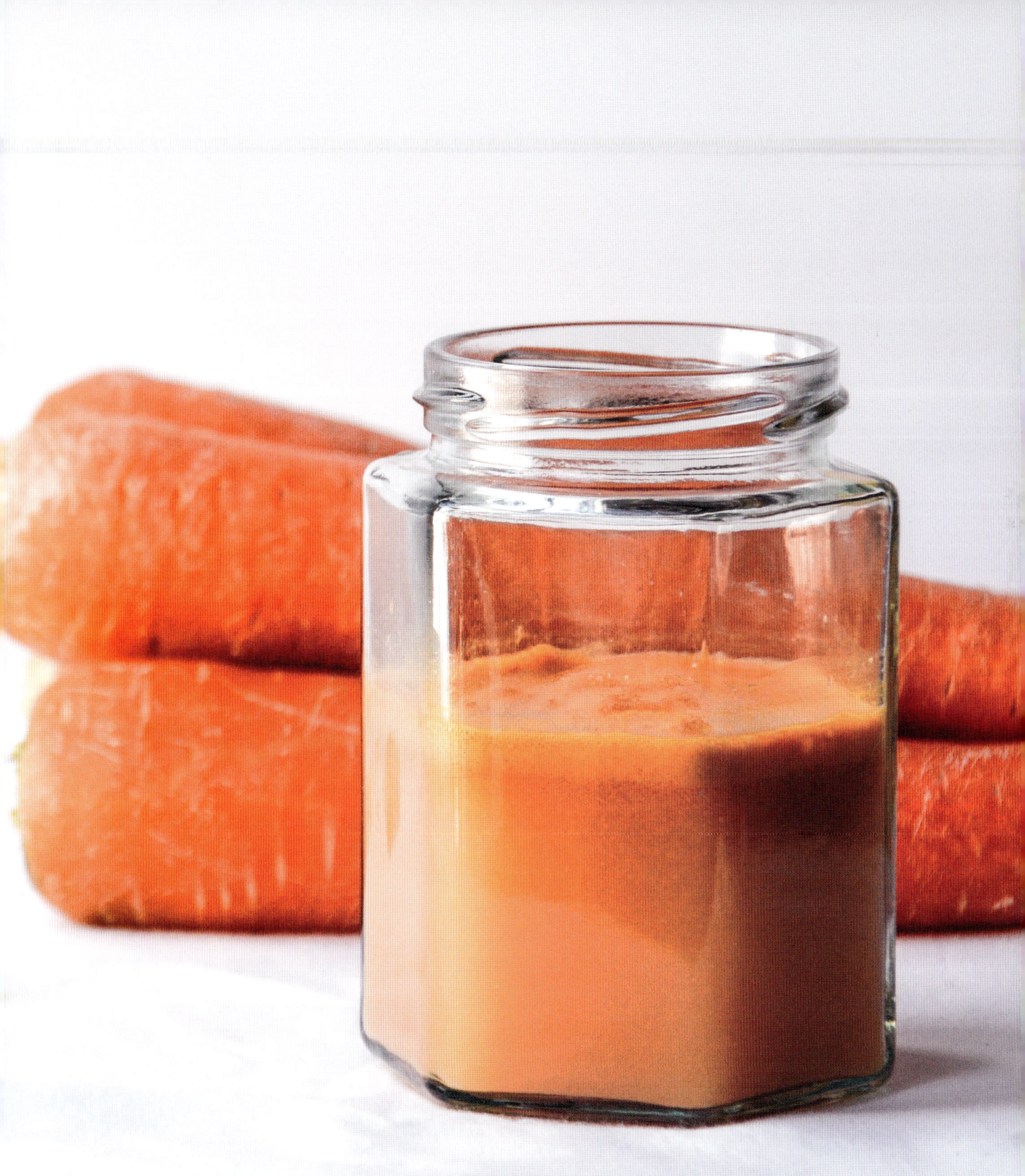

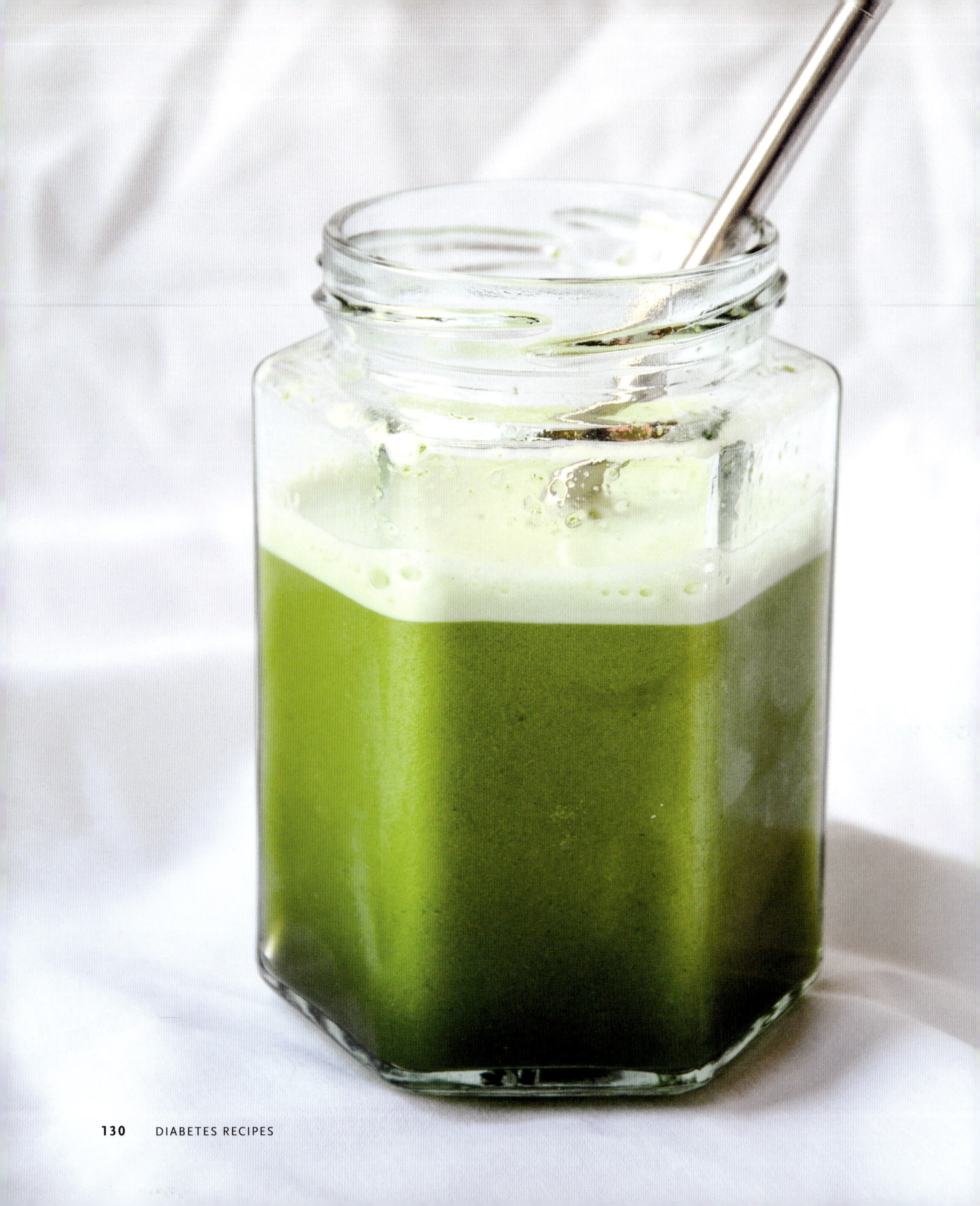

Super greens juice

Green juice trumps all others for health benefits and it's incredibly easy to balance the earthiness of the green vegetables with the addition of a small apple. This recipe really delivers on the super in its name as it crams in as many green veggies as you can handle. The great thing about this recipe is that it's easily customised to what you like or what you have on hand. It takes a basic green juice and steps it up a notch.

SERVES 2

5 cups (150g) spinach leaves

4 celery stalks, plus leaves

1 inch piece of fresh ginger root

1 large cucumber

1 green apple

1 tsp spirulina

Process the spinach leaves in batches through the feed chute of your blender. Follow with the celery and ginger then the cucumber and apple. Right before serving, stir through the spirulina.

Enjoy fresh juice within two hours of making it, if not drinking immediately store the juice in a sealed jar or bottle in the fridge for up to two days.

Lemon, lime + ACV

This zesty juice is a fantastic drink to wake up with in the morning or keep you going in the afternoon. Drinking lemon juice or apple cider vinegar (ACV) first thing in the morning is a great way to kick start digestion and cleanse. Apple cider vinegar is high in acetic acid, a potent antimicrobial that can kill bacteria. It's also a great blood glucose stabiliser and has been shown to improve insulin sensitivity when taken during a meal.

SERVES 1

1 small lemon, peeled

1 lime, peeled

1 large cucumber

2 celery sticks, with leaves

1–2 tbsp apple cider vinegar

Juice the lemon, lime, cucumber and celery sticks together then stir through the apple cider vinegar immediately before drinking.

Want another reason to add apple cider vinegar to your shopping list? It also makes a fantastic beauty tonic, applied topically it can be used as a toner or hair conditioner.

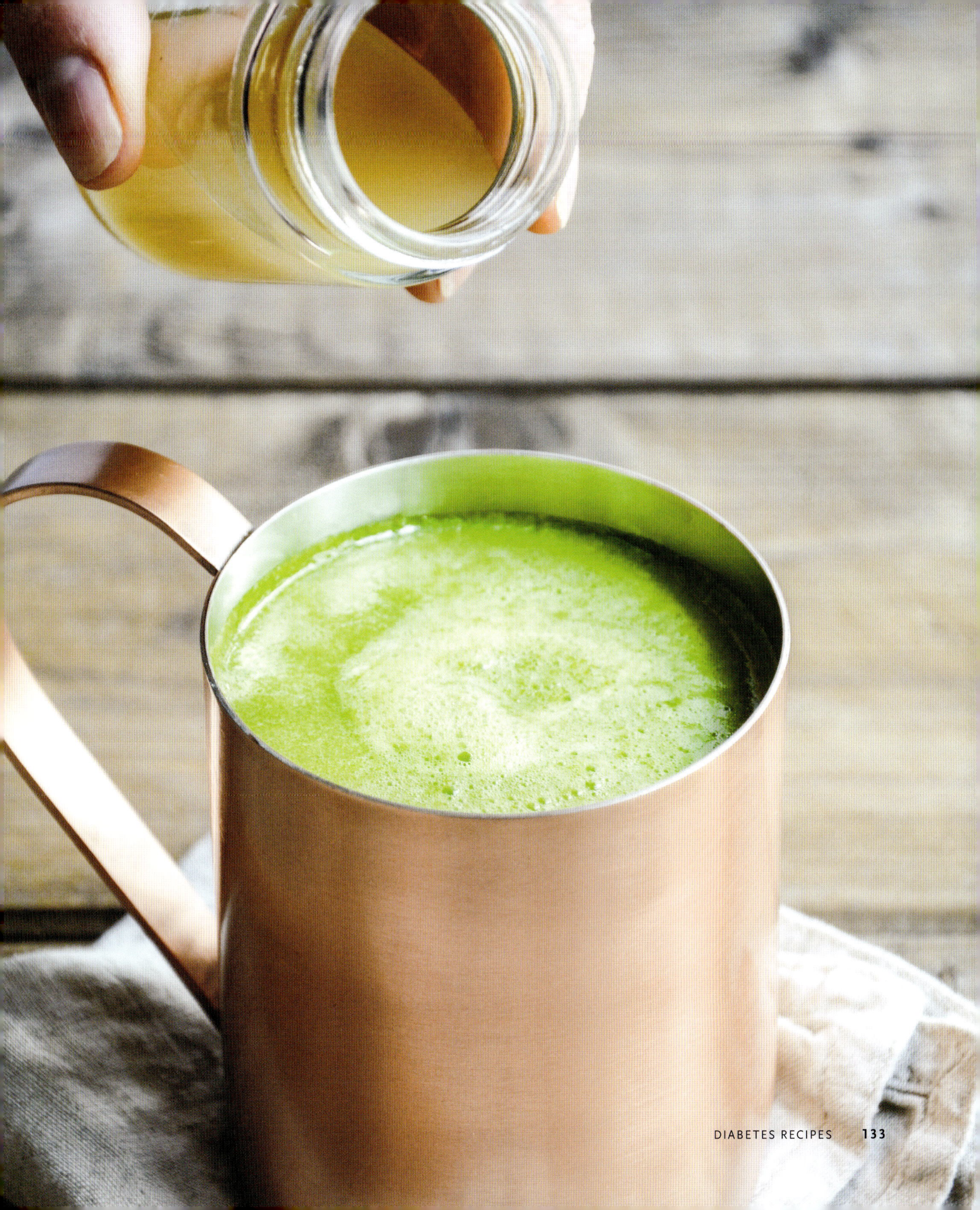

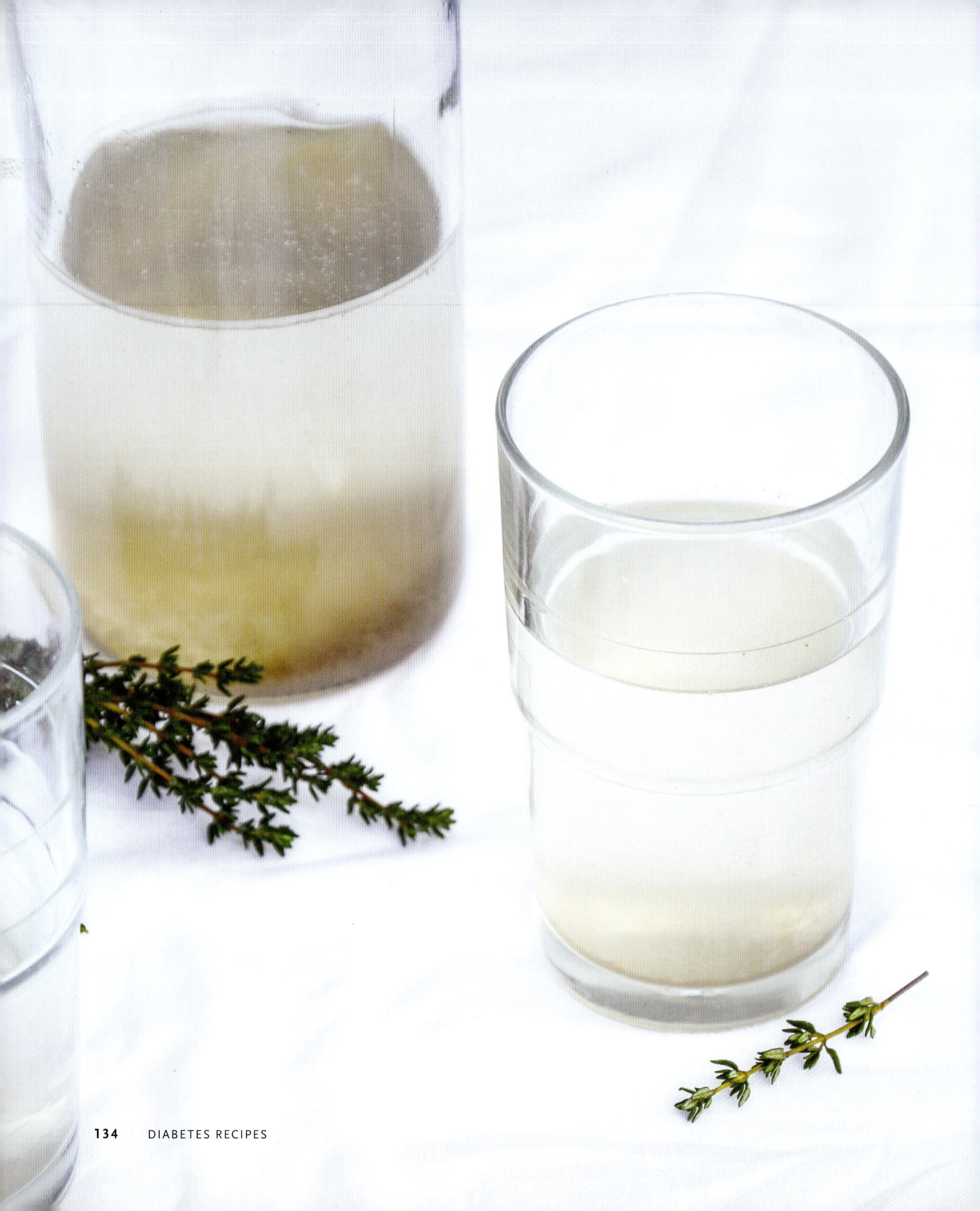

Ginger + lemon thyme fizz

This sweet, natural alternative to soft drink and soda is a real crowd-pleaser. Refreshing in warmer months served with plenty of ice in chilled glasses, or served as the seasons drift into cooler temperatures, with the ginger providing some much-needed warmth; this fizz is a simple syrup that can be mixed with still, sparkling or coconut water.

SERVES 6

150g/5.3 oz fresh ginger root

2 tbsp raw honey

Large handful of fresh lemon thyme sprigs (up to 1 bunch)

1 cup (250ml) water

Still, sparkling or coconut water to serve

1 Prepare the ginger by slicing it into even chunks. You can leave the skin on, however remove any dirty looking bits before adding everything to a small saucepan.

2 Add the honey, lemon thyme sprigs and water, stir then leave to simmer for 30 minutes. Check the liquid level periodically, topping up if it is getting too low. You want the syrup to be concentrated but not too thick.

3 Pour the syrup through a sieve into a jar or jug. When ready to serve, divide the syrup evenly between glasses and top up with still, sparkling or coconut water.

Nut + oat milks

Making milk, sometimes called mylk, from nuts and oats is a popular option for vegans, lactose intolerant people or those who prefer not to consume dairy. While you can buy almond milk in most supermarkets now, they can be expensive and often contain unnecessary ingredients, including sugar. It's easy to make your own nut and oak milks at home if you have a blender to do the hard work for you. You can drink nut milk straight or use it in smoothies or in recipes that call for dairy milk. To build a great smoothie add homemade nut or oak milk, fresh fruit and vegetables and a couple of spoonfuls of almond, Brazil and cashew butter (page 141) to a blender.

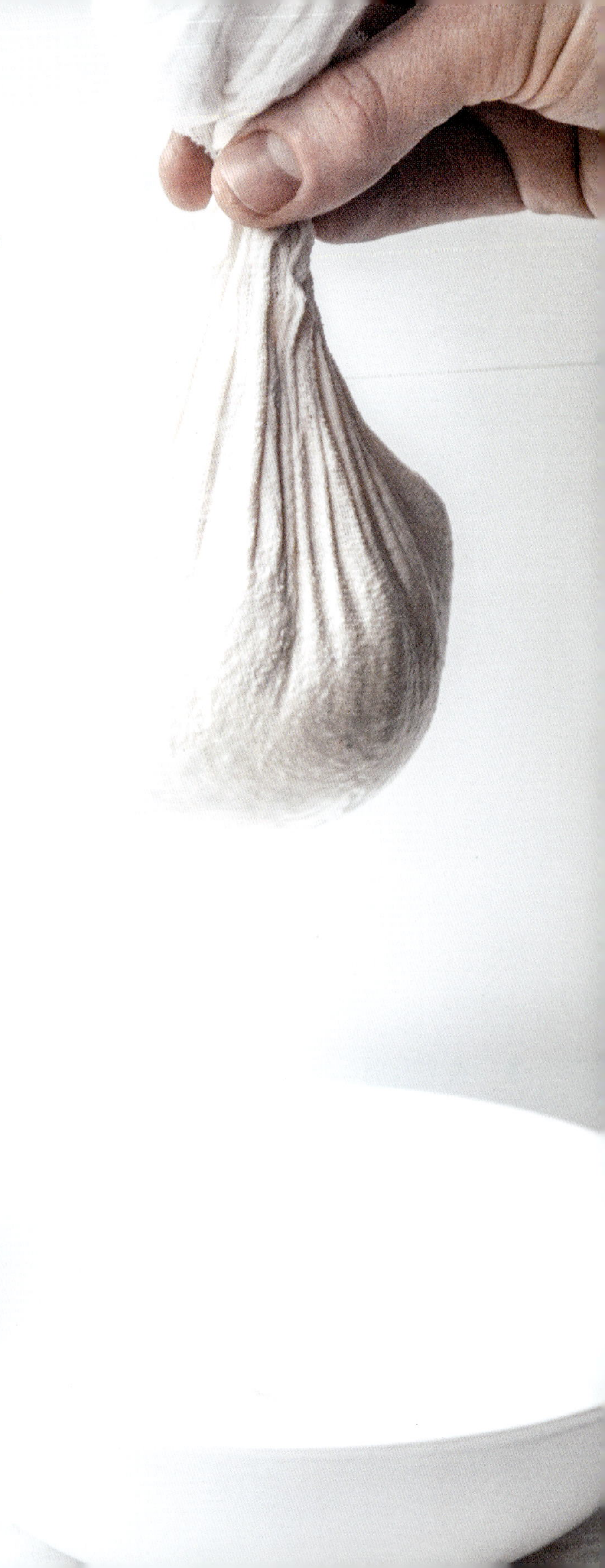

Basic nut milk

Soaking the nuts overnight helps them blend easier and also removes the enzyme inhibitors, phytic acid, polyphenols and goitrogens that coat the nuts. Without soaking, these inhibitors may cause gastrointestinal discomfort such as bloating or gas.

MAKES 4 CUPS/1 LITRE

1½ cups (210g) almonds, cashews, macadamias or Brazil nuts

Water

Optional sweetener such as Medjool dates, maple syrup, rice malt syrup, vanilla powder or cinnamon

1. Soak the nuts overnight in a bowl of filtered water that covers the nuts completely.
2. Rinse the nuts in fresh water, drain then add to a blender with 4 cups (1L) of filtered water. Blend on high until smooth. Place a sieve over a large bowl or jug. Line the sieve with a piece of muslin cloth and pour the nut milk through the cloth to separate the pulp from the milk. Squeeze the pulp in the cloth to drain as much liquid as possible.
3. The nut pulp can be dehydrated into nut meal or can be added to smoothies or sent to the compost heap.
4. If you would like to sweeten the nut milk, blend the sweetener of choice into the strained milk before storing in an airtight jar or container in the fridge. Nut milk is usually good for up to five days.

Oat milk

Oat milk is high in fibre, folic acid and vitamin E. It is not as high in protein as cow's milk is so if you're using it in a smoothie simply add a heaped spoonful of tahini for a nut-free protein boost.

MAKES 4 CUPS/1 LITRE

1½ cups (120g) rolled oats (not quick oats)

Water

Optional sweetener such as Medjool dates, maple syrup, rice malt syrup, vanilla powder or cinnamon

1. Soak the oats in a bowl of filtered water for 1 hour before draining through a sieve, rinsing with fresh water and adding to a blender with 4 cups (1L) of filtered water. Blend on high until smooth.
2. Place a sieve over a large bowl or jug. Line the sieve with a piece of muslin cloth and pour the milk through the cloth to separate the pulp from the milk. Squeeze the pulp in the cloth to drain as much liquid as possible. Discard the oat pulp in the compost heap or bin.

If adding a sweetener, blend the strained milk with sweetener of choice before storing the milk in an airtight container in the fridge for up to five days.

Coconut milk

Coconut milk is a great dairy-free milk to add to your smoothies not only for taste and texture but for nutritional benefits also. It's packed with healthy fats to keep you feeling full for longer, while the oil in the coconut milk helps boost metabolism. The lauric acid in coconuts is thought to help the body fight off infections and viruses, and the high levels of minerals including selenium, calcium and magnesium further boost its nutritional profile.

MAKES 1½ CUPS/375ML

2 cups (500ml) filtered water

1 cup (110g) unsweetened shredded coconut or coconut chips

1 Heat the water in a saucepan to a simmer then pour into the blender carefully. Add the shredded coconut and place the lid on the blender, blend for one minute on low before increasing the speed to medium for a further minute. Increase the speed to high for one minute until smooth and creamy.

2 Line a bowl with a fine mesh sieve or a piece of muslin cloth. Pour the coconut milk through the sieve or cloth to remove any remaining piece of coconut. If using a sieve, use the back of a spoon to push down and press out as much liquid as you can. If using muslin cloth, bring the sides of the cloth together so the pulp is inside and squeeze with your hands to extract any remaining liquid.

3 Store in an airtight jar or container in the fridge for up to five days.

Pina colada

Yes, if you like pina coladas and getting caught in the rain then you're sure to enjoy this real food spin on the classic cocktail.

SERVES 1

1 cup (250ml) coconut milk

4 ice cubes

200g/7 oz fresh pineapple

1 tsp ground cinnamon

½ tsp ground nutmeg

⅓ cup (80ml) filtered water (optional)

Add the coconut milk and ice cubes to the blender. Chop the pineapple into even-sized chunks and add to the blender with the cinnamon and nutmeg. Blend on high until smooth and creamy. If the smoothie needs to be thinned down add the filtered water and blend for 20 seconds.

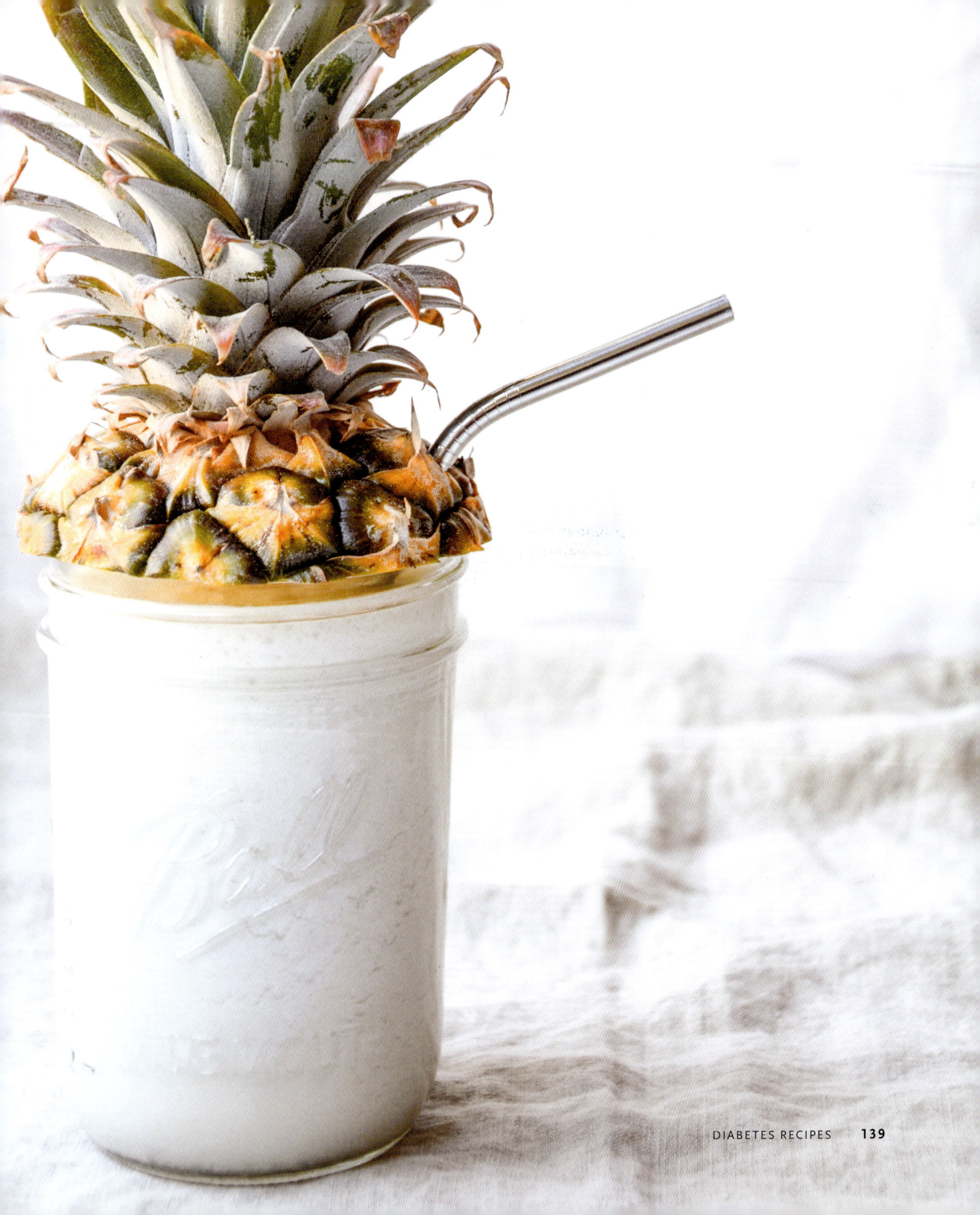

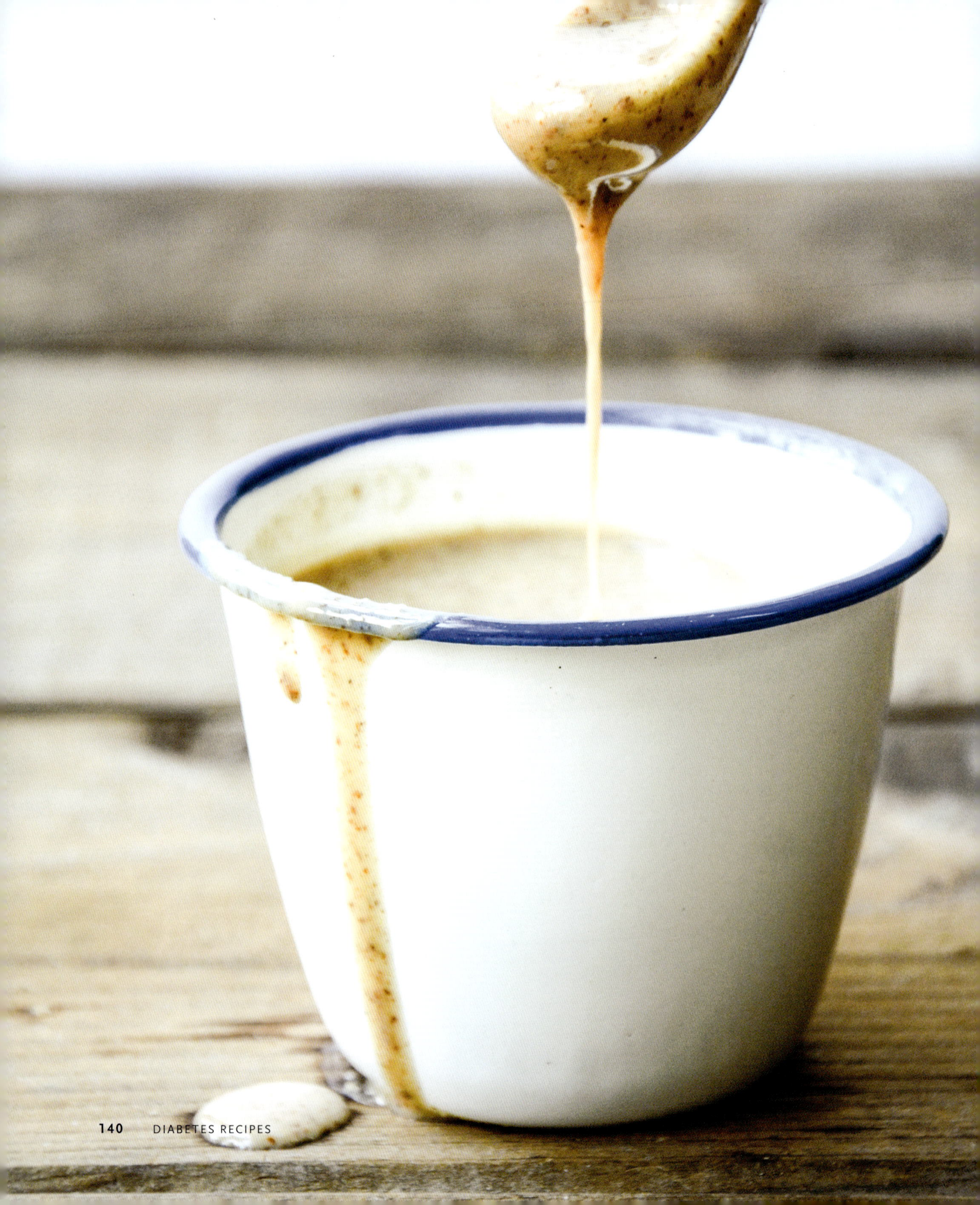

Almond, Brazil + cashew butter

This is a classic three-nut butter blend commonly referred to as ABC butter, I think you can figure out why. All three nuts are nutrient dense but it's the cashews that make this nut butter particularly creamy. This is great to make ahead and store in an airtight container or jar in the fridge. Simply add a couple of spoonfuls of the butter to your next smoothie for a protein boost.

MAKES 1½ CUPS

1 cup (140g) raw almonds, soaked overnight

1 cup (130g) raw Brazil nuts, soaked overnight

1 cup (110g) raw cashews, soaked overnight

Add the nuts to a blender or the bowl of a food processor fitted with the S blade attachment and blitz on high until a fine crumb forms. Scrape down the sides of the bowl with a spatula and continue blending on high until the butter forms. The time this takes will vary depending on your equipment (it can be anywhere from 10-20 minutes) so have patience. At times it may look like the butter will never come together but it has to get crumbly before it can get smooth, trust me.

Store in an airtight container in the fridge for up to two weeks. If the oils naturally separate simply stir the butter before using.

treats

Goji berry + sea salt truffles
Raw carrot cake slice
Macadamia rock cakes
Baked gingerbread doughnuts with tahini glaze
Zucchini + blueberry tea cake
Chai tea poached peaches with macadamia crumble
Vanilla cupcakes with chocolate frosting
Chickpea chocolate chip cookies
Let's date cake

Goji berry + sea salt truffles

Heaven is surely an unlimited supply of raw chocolate truffles while you lounge about on a fluffy cloud. These truffles are not only quick to make but basically foolproof, meaning you throw everything together in a bowl, stick it in the fridge to harden, then roll into bite-size treats that dreams are made of.

MAKES 12

4 tbsp cacao butter

3 tbsp coconut oil

3 tbsp rice malt syrup, honey or maple syrup

¾ cup (90g) raw cacao powder

1 tsp sea salt

½ cup (55g) goji berries

COATING

⅓ cup (40g) goji berries

¼ cup (20g) unsweetened shredded coconut

1 In a small saucepan melt the cacao butter and coconut oil over a low heat. As soon as the mixture turns liquid remove it from the heat and whisk in your sweetener of choice.

2 Sift in the raw cacao powder and whisk until the mixture is smooth and glossy.

3 Stir through the sea salt and goji berries then pour the mixture into a shallow bowl and place in the refrigerator for 15–20 minutes.

4 While the mixture is cooling, prepare the coating to roll the truffles in. Place the goji berries and coconut in the bowl of a food processor and blitz into a powder. Pour the powder over a large plate and set aside.

5 When the chocolate mixture has begun to harden, take it out of the fridge and use a teaspoon to scoop up small amounts. Roll the chocolate between your palms into a ball shape, working quickly as your body heat will melt the mixture.

6 Place the balls on the plate of goji berry powder, roll to coat the outside then place the truffles in an airtight container and store in the refrigerator for up to 2 weeks.

TRY:

COFFEE + COCONUT

Mix 1 heaped tbsp of coffee granules into the basic truffle mixture (omitting the sea salt and goji berries from the previous recipe) and roll the balls in unsweetened shredded coconut.

BLUEBERRY + GINGER

Mix 1 heaped tbsp of freshly grated ginger and ⅓ cup (50g) of chopped blueberries into the basic truffle mixture and roll the balls in raw cacao powder.

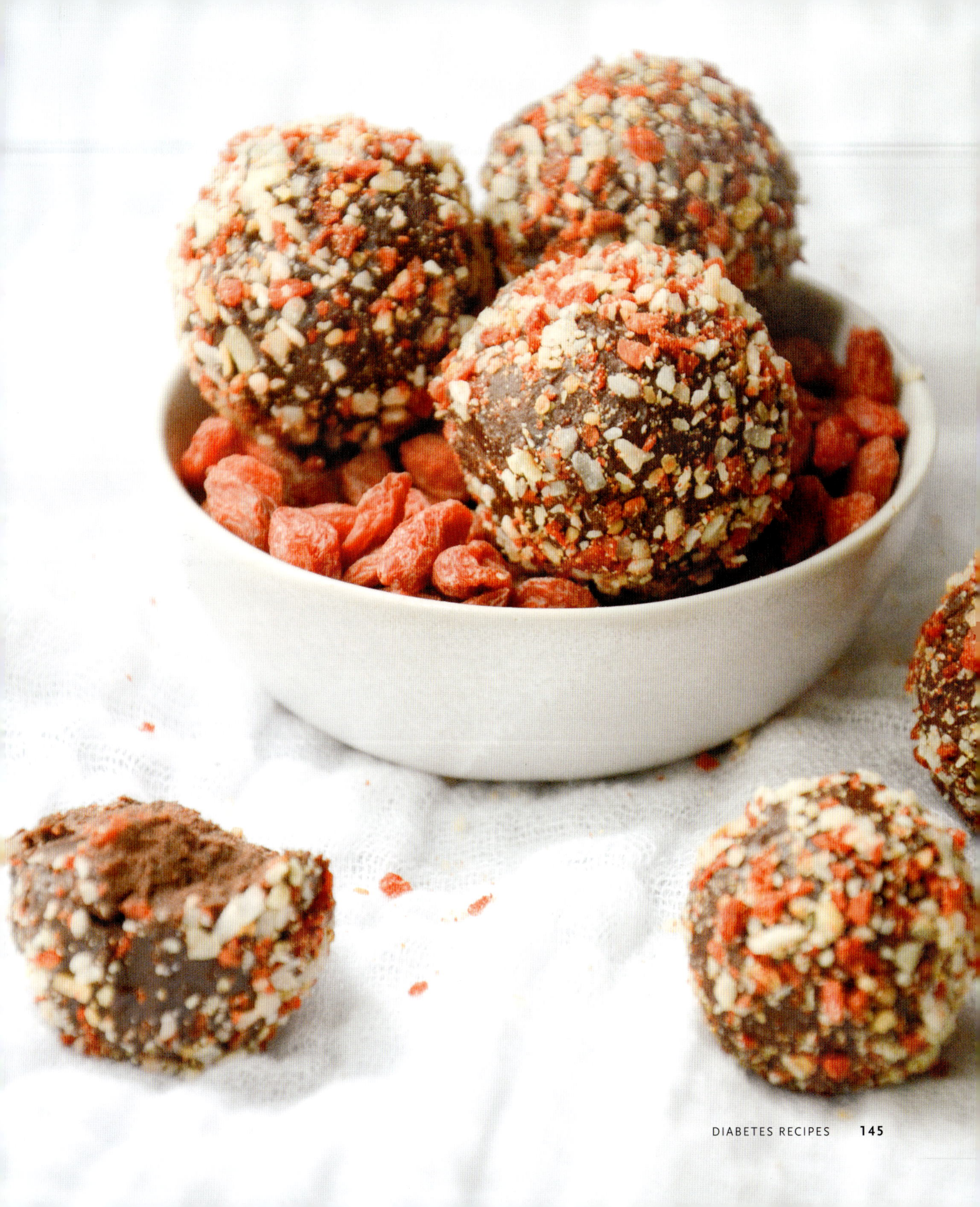

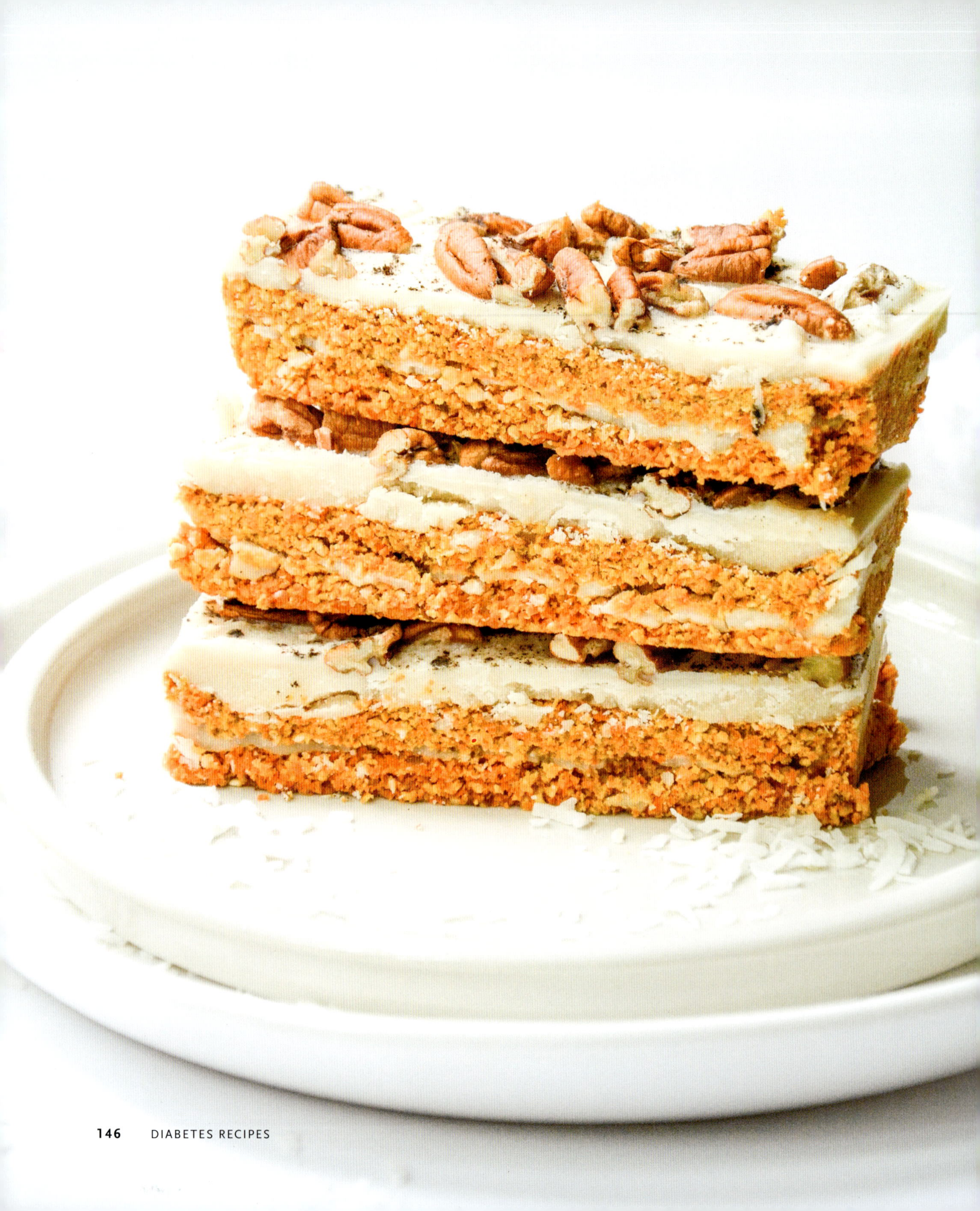

Raw carrot cake slice

Carrot cake is one of those desserts that sounds healthy but is often far from it. Here we replace refined white flour with rolled oats or quinoa flakes, sweeten with dates instead of white sugar, and top the cake off with an indulgent coconut butter frosting instead of cream cheese. The earthy flavour of the raw carrots still shines through and is not masked by the other ingredients, making this a real treat for those who love the taste of their vegetables.

SERVES 8

6 Medjool dates, pitted

3 large carrots, peeled

1 cup (100g) rolled oats or quinoa flakes

½ cup (85g) pecans

¾ cup (60g) unsweetened shredded coconut

1 tsp ground cinnamon

½ tsp ground nutmeg

FROSTING

1 cup (230g) coconut butter

1 cup (250ml) melted coconut oil

⅓ cup (80ml) rice malt syrup or maple syrup

Vanilla powder and extra pecans for decorating

1 Soak the dates in a bowl of boiling water while you prepare the cake mixture.

2 Peel the carrots and chop into small chunks. Place in the bowl of a food processor along with the oats, pecans, coconut, cinnamon and nutmeg. Blitz until the mixture forms a fine crumb and the carrot is evenly distributed.

3 Drain the dates from the water and remove the pits. Place the dates in the bowl of the food processor and pulse the mixture until mixed with the carrot.

4 Line a rectangular or square baking tin with baking paper and press half of the carrot mixture into the tin, pushing it down firmly.

5 Prepare the frosting by adding the coconut butter, coconut oil and sweetener of choice to the bowl of a food processor and blitzing until smooth.

6 Spread ⅓ of the frosting mixture over the carrot mixture in the tin, smooth out into each corner with a knife. Place in the refrigerator for 5 minutes for the frosting to harden.

7 Press the rest of the carrot cake mixture into the tin then spread the remaining coconut frosting over the top, sprinkle with a pinch of vanilla powder and a small handful of chopped pecans.

8 Set in the refrigerator for 20 minutes, slice into bars or squares and store in an airtight container in the fridge.

Macadamia rock cakes

Consider making these in mini muffin tins or muffin liners for a bite-size treat. With a rich coconut flavour and a hit of raw chocolate on the top, these rock cakes are sure to curb any cravings you may encounter after dinner.

MAKES 6

1½ cups (225g) macadamia nuts
1 cup (80g) shredded coconut
3 tbsp coconut butter
1 tsp sea salt
¼ cup (60ml) rice malt syrup

CHOCOLATE TOPPING

¼ cup (60ml) coconut oil, melted
¼ cup (30g) raw cacao powder
Pinch of sea salt
1 tbsp rice malt syrup

1 Place the macadamia nuts in a food processor and pulse until crumbs form. Add the coconut, coconut butter, salt and rice malt syrup and pulse until combined. Press spoonfuls of the mixture into 6 holes of a muffin tin. Keep adding mixture until all used and press down hard. You can also make these in baking cups or using muffin liners. Place the tin in the refrigerator for 1 hour until the cakes have firmed up.

2 Prepare the chocolate topping by combining the coconut oil, raw cacao, sea salt and rice malt syrup. Stir or whisk until smooth.

3 Take the rock cakes out of the refrigerator and use a butter knife to help ease them out of the tin. Dip the top of each cake into the chocolate mixture and turn to drain the excess. Place on a plate ready to eat or store in the fridge.

Raw cacao is loaded with magnesium, which can help regulate mood and reduce stress and sugar cravings. It also raises serotonin levels and doesn't contribute to insulin spikes. Raw cacao is available in specialty grocers and health food stores and boasts a higher nutrient content than regular cocoa.

Baked gingerbread doughnuts with tahini glaze

Baked doughnuts are a revelation in home cooked delights. Of course they'll never be as mouth watering as the deep fried versions but these can be enjoyed more regularly without having to undo the top button on your pants afterwards. Pairing gingerbread with a tahini glaze may sound a little strange to some people but it is worth trying at least once. The spiciness of the gingerbread is mellowed by the nutty tahini and it's surprising how well they compliment each other.

MAKES 8

1 cup (130g) brown rice flour
1 tsp baking powder
½ tsp ground cinnamon
1½ tsp ground ginger
Pinch of sea salt
1 tbsp coconut oil, melted
1 free range egg
2 tbsp milk
1 tsp molasses (optional)
1 tbsp maple or rice malt syrup

TAHINI GLAZE

½ cup (115g) hulled tahini
1 tbsp maple syrup
Pinch of sea salt

1 Preheat the oven to 180°C/350°F.

2 Sift the rice flour, baking powder, cinnamon, ginger and sea salt into a bowl.

3 In a separate bowl whisk the coconut oil, egg, milk, molasses (if using) and maple syrup together then stir through the flour mix. Transfer the batter to a piping bag (or use a ziplock bag and snip the end off) and pipe the mixture into 6 holes of a doughnut pan, careful not to overfill the holes as the batter will rise considerably.

4 Bake the doughnuts in the oven for 15–20 minutes until golden brown, the doughnuts should feel light and an inserted skewer should come out clean. Remove the doughnuts from the pan and cool on a wire rack.

5 Prepare the glaze by adding the tahini, maple syrup and sea salt to a bowl and whisking until smooth, adding a dash of water if the glaze needs thinning out.

6 Once the doughnuts have cooled down, spread 1 tbsp of glaze onto each and enjoy. Store any leftovers in an airtight container to be eaten within 2 days.

Zucchini + blueberry tea cake

This barely sweet tea cake earns its name because it goes perfectly with a freshly brewed cup of tea. The addition of zucchini keeps the cake moist while the blueberries deliver pockets of sweetness and tartness, while also giving the cake a beautiful colour. I love to eat this fresh from the oven, warm with a smear of soft grass fed butter.

SERVES 8

3 free range eggs

1 cup (250ml) coconut oil, melted

½ cup (125ml) milk of choice

½ cup (125ml) rice malt syrup or sweetener of choice

1 tsp vanilla powder

1 large zucchini/courgette

1½ cups (195g) brown rice flour

1 cup (120g) buckwheat flour

2 tsp baking powder

Pinch of sea salt

200g/7 oz blueberries, fresh or frozen

1 Preheat the oven to 180°C/350°F and line a loaf tin with baking paper.

2 In a medium bowl whisk the eggs with the melted coconut oil, milk, sweetener and vanilla powder. Grate the zucchini and add to the wet mixture, stir until combined.

3 Sift in the rice and buckwheat flours along with the baking powder and salt. Fold through the blueberries then pour the batter into the lined loaf tin. Bake in the oven for 40 minutes or until an inserted skewer comes out clean.

4 Remove from the pan and let the cake rest on a wire rack for 10 minutes. Serve warm or cold as is or with a smear of butter.

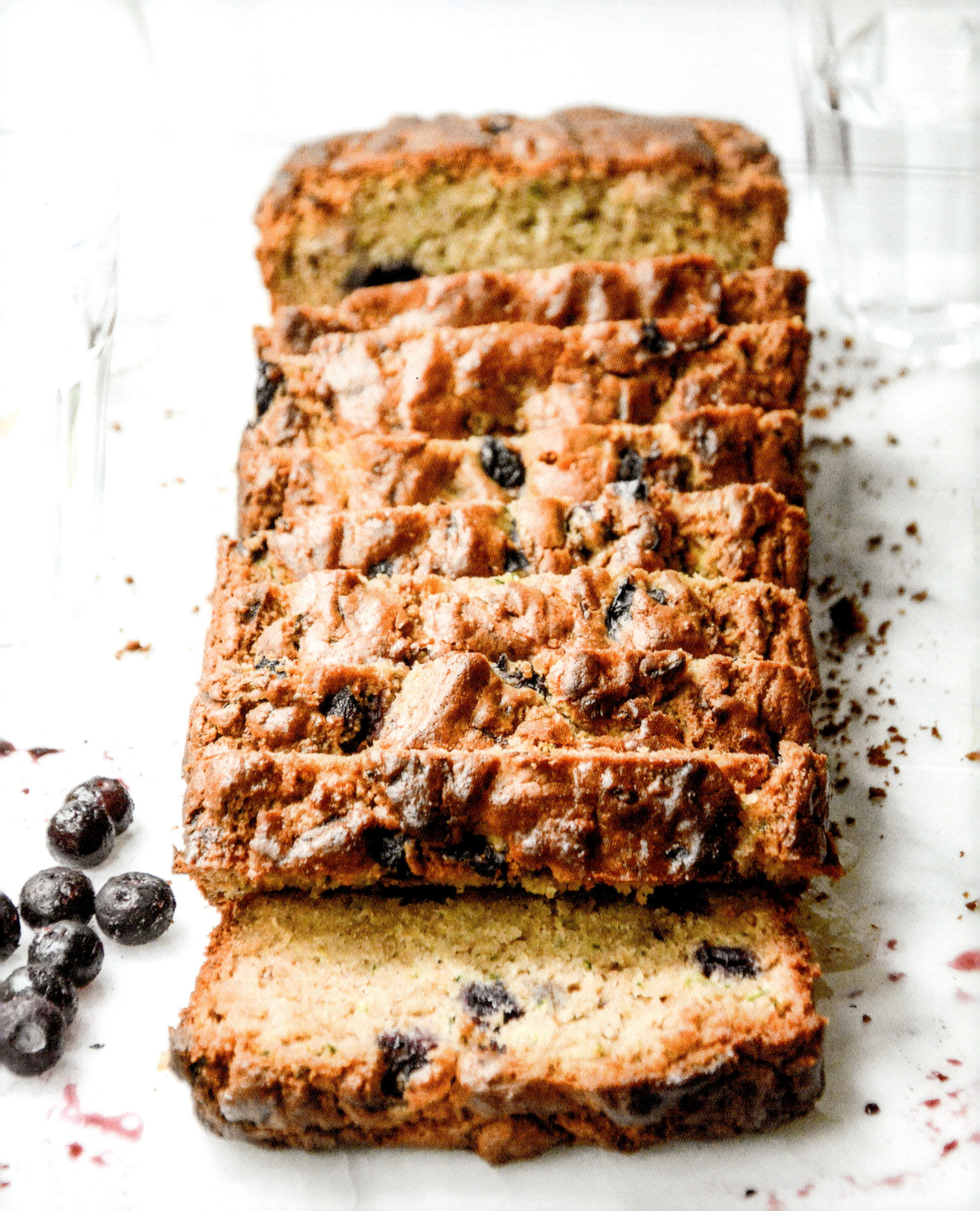

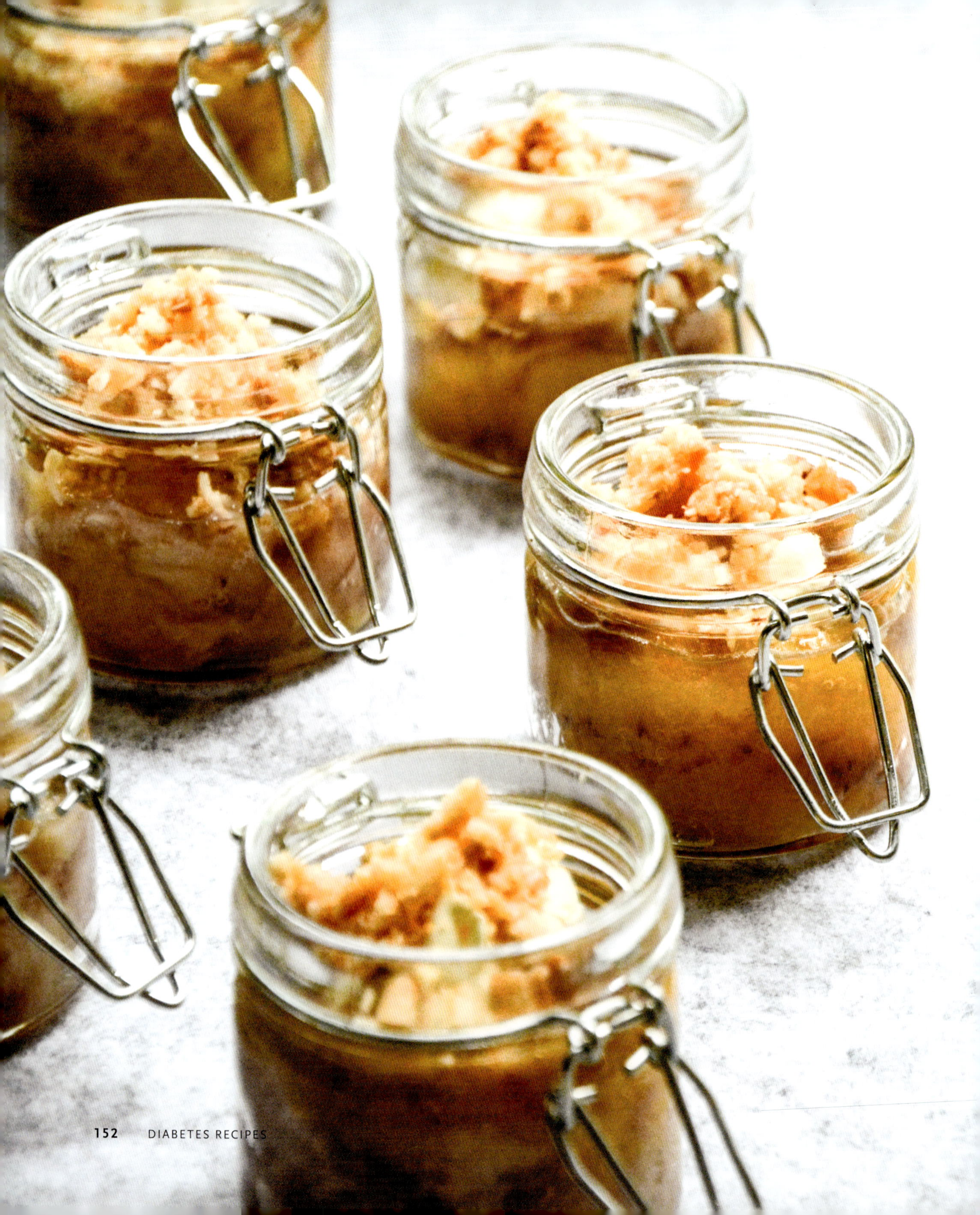

Chai tea poached peaches with macadamia crumble

You can make one large crumble with this recipe or serve in individual pots, which works great for a party. The poached peaches can be served warm or chilled, depending on the occasion. These are great to make ahead of time and store in the refrigerator for up to three days, and of course the peaches can be substituted with any stone fruit of choice.

SERVES 6

2 tbsp loose chai tea leaves/mix

6 cups (1.5L) filtered water

6 peaches

1 cup (150g) macadamia nuts

½ cup (40g) unsweetened shredded coconut

25g/1 oz grass fed butter

1 tsp ground cinnamon

1 Add the tea and water to a saucepan over medium heat and let it simmer for 5 minutes to brew.

2 Cut a cross into the top of each peach then lower them gently into the water. If the water doesn't cover the peaches, top the pan up with a little extra water. Poach the peaches in the tea for 30 minutes until tender then remove the pan from the heat and place in the fridge for anywhere from 1 hour to overnight to let the flavour intensify.

3 Peel the skin off the peaches and cut or pull the peaches into chunks. Evenly distribute the peaches between jars or bowls and prepare the macadamia crumble.

4 Preheat the oven to 180°C/350°F. In the bowl of a food processor fitted with an S blade blitz the macadamia nuts, coconut, butter and cinnamon until a crumb forms. Spread the crumb over an oven tray lined with baking paper and bake for 15 minutes or until the mixture has browned.

5 Sprinkle the macadamia crumble over the top of the poached peaches and serve.

Poaching the fruit in tea removes the need for adding sweetener to the recipe and allows you to infuse a range of flavours into the peaches. Try experimenting with different tea and fruit combinations. If you cannot source loose leaf tea, simply use tea bags that you have on hand.

Vanilla cupcakes with chocolate frosting

There's no need to remove cake entirely from your life if you're prepared to think outside the box a little. These vanilla cupcakes are wheat free and use coconut flour, creating a light and fluffy texture. Rice malt syrup is used instead of white refined sugar, which should help to reduce the likelihood of spiking blood glucose levels. As with any sweet recipe, these are best shared around and portion control is advised.

MAKES 12

½ cup (125ml) coconut butter, melted

1½ cups (375ml) coconut milk

½ cup (125ml) rice malt syrup

1 vanilla bean pod

6 free range eggs

¾ cup (100g) coconut flour

CHOCOLATE FROSTING

3 tbsp coconut oil, melted

3 tbsp coconut milk

3 tbsp maple syrup or sweetener of choice

3 tbsp raw cacao powder

1 tbsp Dutch press cocoa

¼ tsp vanilla powder

Fresh fruit, nuts, seeds or coconut to decorate

1 Preheat the oven to 160°C/320°F.

2 In a saucepan combine the coconut butter, coconut milk and rice malt syrup together with the seeds from the vanilla bean pod. Take off the heat and set aside.

3 Separate the egg yolks and whites. Whisk the whites to stiff peaks and set aside. Stir the egg yolks through the cooled coconut mixture followed by the coconut flour.

4 Fold the whipped egg whites through the mixture until just combined, taking care not to lose too much air from the mixture.

5 Use an ice cream scoop to evenly distribute the batter between 12 cupcake liners and bake in the oven for 30 minutes or until an inserted skewer comes out clean. Remove from the oven and cool on a wire rack.

6 Prepare the frosting by whisking together the coconut oil, coconut milk, rice malt syrup, raw cacao powder, Dutch press cocoa and vanilla powder until smooth and glossy. Dip each cupcake into the frosting and turn to allow the excess to drip off. Alternatively, place the frosting in the fridge for 5 minutes to firm up then spread over the top of the cupcakes. Top each cupcake with your fruit of choice, such as pomegranate seeds or orange segments, shredded coconut or chopped nuts.

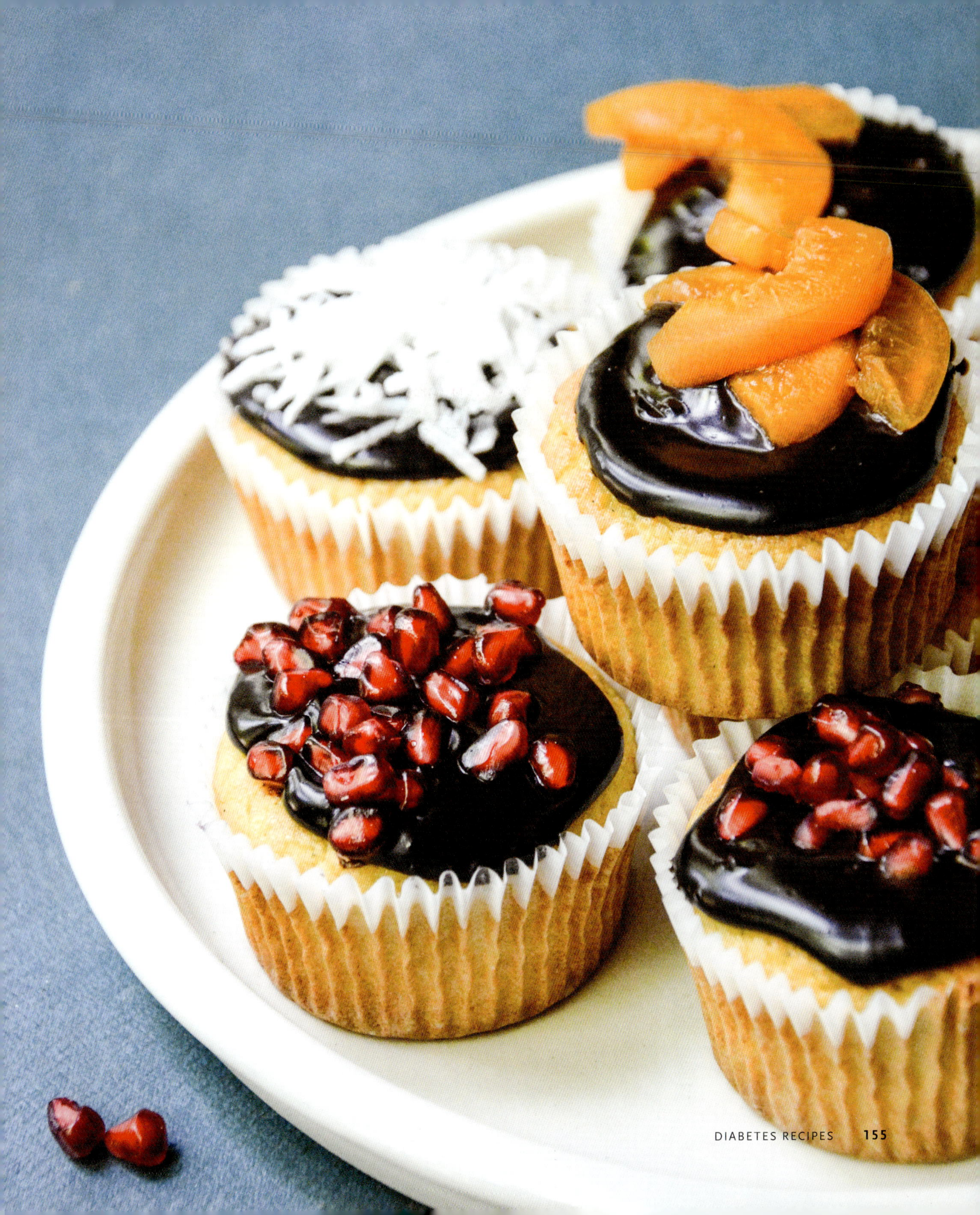

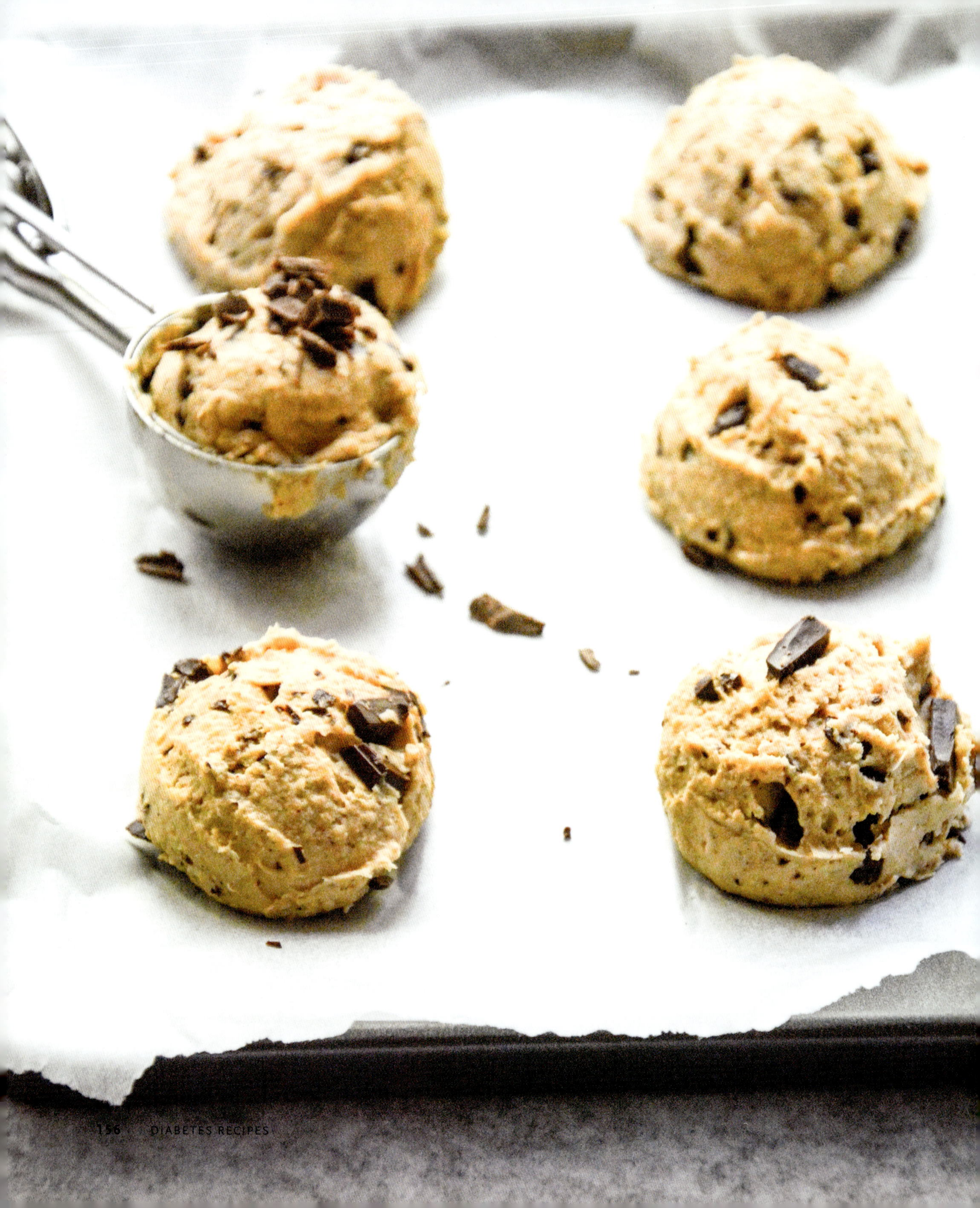

Chickpea chocolate chip cookies

The sweetness in this recipe comes from the dark chocolate, use only the best quality and the darker the better. If you'd rather omit the chocolate, you can add chopped walnuts or cacao nibs for something different. If using either of these you may want to add a small amount of sweetener to the dough such as rice malt syrup, maple syrup or raw honey. As these cookies don't have the amount of sugars, stabilisers or artificial ingredients as store-bought cookies their shelf life is considerably less. Bake cookies as needed and freeze the rest of the dough.

MAKES 12

400g/14 oz cooked chickpeas

⅔ cup (90g) brown rice flour

1 tsp baking powder

⅓ cup (80ml) coconut oil, melted

2 tbsp milk (nut milk can be substituted)

1 tsp vanilla powder

1 tsp cinnamon

1 tsp nutmeg

2 tsp sea salt

⅔ cup (170g) dark chocolate chips

1 Preheat the oven to 180°C/350°F.

2 Rinse and drain the chickpeas from the can then add to the bowl of a food processor fitted with the S blade attachment. Puree until smooth then add the flour and baking powder and pulse.

3 Scrape down the sides of the bowl then add the coconut oil, milk, vanilla powder, cinnamon, nutmeg and sea salt. Pulse until combined. Stir through the chocolate chips.

4 Roll the dough into small balls or use an ice cream scoop to create even-sized cookies and then place on an oven tray lined with baking paper. Use the back of a fork to press each ball down slightly. Bake for 20 minutes then set on a wire rack to cool slightly and firm up. Store in an airtight container.

Let's date cake

This moist date and coconut cake is a great special occasion recipe when you want a sweet indulgence that's tasty but easy to whip up. You can top the cake with the coconut frosting or regular cream, or simply enjoy it frosting free with fresh berries on the side.

SERVES 8

250g/9 oz fresh Medjool dates, pitted

1 cup (80g) shredded coconut

½ cup (125ml) melted butter

½ cup (125ml) coconut milk

5 free range eggs, separated

¾ cup (75g) almond meal

1 tsp ground cinnamon

1 tsp ground ginger

1 tsp vanilla powder

COCONUT FROSTING

1 cup (250ml) coconut milk, refrigerated overnight

Pinch of vanilla powder

1 Preheat the oven to 170°C/320°F. Grease one large spring form tin with butter and place a circle of greaseproof paper on the bottom of the tin (to help remove the cake easier when cooked).

2 Blitz the dates and shredded coconut in a food processor before adding the melted butter and coconut milk.

3 Using a stand mixer or a handheld mixer beat the egg yolks with the cinnamon, ginger and vanilla until just thicker in consistency, approximately 2–4 minutes.

4 In a large mixing bowl combine the egg yolk mixture with the date mixture then stir the almond meal through gently.

5 Beat the egg whites in a clean bowl until stiff peaks form. Fold the beaten egg whites gently through the rest of the mixture.

6 Pour the batter into the prepared tin and bake in the oven for 35–45 minutes or until an inserted skewer comes out clean. Once cooked, let cool for 10 minutes in the tin before turning out onto a wire rack and leaving to cool completely.

7 Prepare the whipped coconut frosting by whisking (either by hand or using a stand mixer) the coconut milk with a pinch of vanilla powder until thickened. It's best to refrigerate the coconut milk overnight to help it thicken when whisking, however refrigerating for a period of four hours or more will also help. You can replace the coconut milk with unsweetened whipped cream if desired.

8 Pour the frosting over the cake and garnish with fresh strawberries.

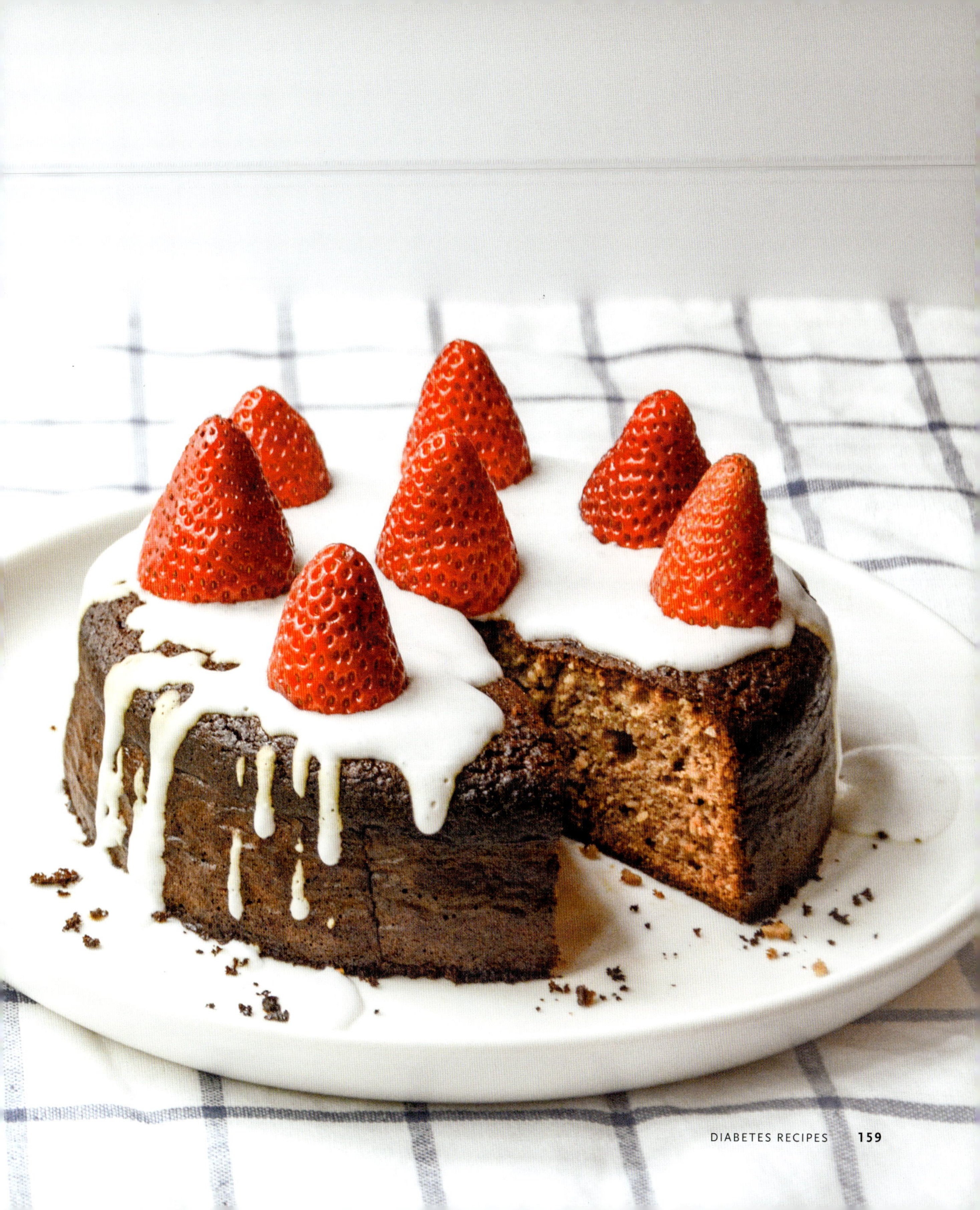

Recipe index

BREAKFAST

Wok eggs with fresh greens 36
Sweet potato + bacon muffins 37
Sprouted lentil + artichoke bowl 38
Strawberry chia pudding 41
Pumpkin pie chia pudding 42
Brunch salad 45
Potato + leek hash browns 47
Super citrus granola with poached pear 48
Triple berry quinoa porridge 50

SALADS & SIDES

Carrot + black sesame salad 54
Choose your greens salad 54
Garlic stir fried broccoli + green beans 56
Fresh freekeh salad 59
Roasted Brussels sprouts with tahini dressing 60
Simple tuna salad 63
Avocado, haloumi + raspberry salad 64
Simple coleslaw 64
Cauliflower tabouli 67
Chilli pumpkin + goat cheese spread 68
Zucchini hummus 70
Lemon hummus 70
Avocado white bean smash 71
Baba ganoush dip 71
Basic sauerkraut 72
Simple kim chi 75
Peach, prosciutto + goat cheese rolls 76
Pepita crusted chicken strips 79
Potato wedges with guacamole 80
Prawn + sprouts rice paper rolls 83

MAINS

Lemon lentil soup 87
Cauliflower + horseradish soup 88
Beef bone broth 91
Spicy beef + Tuscan kale stew 92
Potato + snow pea green curry 95
Quinoa "fried rice" 96
Herbed mushrooms on socca 99
Sweet potato, black bean + jalapeno burger patties 100
Pulled cider pork with roasted garlic + apple salad 102
Chicken + avocado skewers 103
Sweet potato noodle stir-fry 104
Roast paprika chicken 106
Dukkah crusted chicken maryland with confetti rice 109
Cashew satay beef skewers 110
Meatball subs with tomato relish 113
Spring vegetable instant noodle pot 115
Creamy mushroom instant noodle pot 115
Pan seared salmon with dill pea mash 116
Veg packed bolognaise 119

DRINKS

Cucumber chia smoothie 123
Coconut + cucumber lemonade 123
Choc malt cacao nib crunch 124
Golden turmeric milk 127
Turmeric + carrot juice 128
Super greens juice 131
Lemon, lime + ACV 132
Ginger + lemon thyme fizz 135
Basic nut milk 137
Oat milk 137
Coconut milk 138
Pina colada 138
Almond, Brazil and cashew butter 141

TREATS

Goji berry + sea salt truffles 144
Raw carrot cake slice 147
Macadamia rock cakes 148
Baked gingerbread doughnuts with tahini glaze 149
Zucchini + blueberry tea cake 150
Chai tea poached peaches with macadamia crumble 153
Vanilla cupcakes with chocolate frosting 154
Chickpea chocolate chip cookies 157
Let's date cake 158